# Reverberations of a Stroke

Karl Gustafson

# Reverberations of a Stroke

## A Memoir

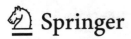 Springer

Karl Gustafson
Department of Mathematics
University of Colorado
Boulder, CO, USA

ISBN 978-3-030-12864-7          ISBN 978-3-030-12862-3    (eBook)
https://doi.org/10.1007/978-3-030-12862-3

Library of Congress Control Number: 2019934351

This Springer imprint is published by the registered company Springer Nature Switzerland AG
The registered company address is: Gewerbestrasse 11, 6330 Cham, Switzerland

*The physicist Leo Szilard once announced to his friend Hans Bethe that he was thinking of keeping a diary. 'I don't intend to publish. I am merely going to record the facts for the information of God.'*

*'Don't you think God knows the facts?' Bethe asked.*

*'Yes,' said Szilard. 'He knows the facts, but He does not know this version of the facts.'*
Hans Christian van Baeyer, *Taming the Atom*
*(Random House, 1992)*

# Foreword by Simo Puntanen: *Eight Months Before a Second Life...*

It was a dark and stormy night.

> Subject: China, Southern provinces: Maintain flexible itineraries due to potential for disruption to flights, overland travel during rainy season—Disruption to travel and essential services should be expected in the southern provinces during the rainy season. Hundreds of flights were canceled or delayed on 2 June at Shanghai Pudong International Airport due to poor weather conditions.

I received the above emailed message from Karl Gustafson on Wednesday, June 3, 2015, with the following line: "Maybe we were lucky to get up here from Haikou Sunday night, even if very late! Karl."

Karl was not joking, and I, being from the largest Nordic city without access to the sea, from a city of the most reserved and introverted people of Finland, never make jokes.

We were in Haikou on May 31, 2015, seven of us from around the world who were headed to *The Second Shanghai Forum of Trade and Financial Statistics* (SFTFS-2015), which would begin the next day. Our original plan was to fly earlier in the day from Haikou to Shanghai Pudong on China Southern Airlines CZ6765. However, already in March, our flight had been rescheduled to leave two hours later than planned, bringing us to our hotels rather late at night. On Sunday, in good time, our team was sitting in two limos, ready to leave Haikou's Ming Guang International Grand Hotel for the Haikou Airport. But when we arrived at the airport, nothing happened. Nothing except hours of waiting. The weather simply would not cooperate.

Finally sometime after midnight, our Airbus A320 was ready to take off, leading to a three-hour very bumpy flight. Otherwise without incident, we arrived in Shanghai, met by our guides. But then, it turned out that they had forgotten where in the parking garage their bus, coming for us, had been left parked. After some time solving that mystery, we finally headed off for the International Exchange Center Hotel, where we would be staying during the conference. We did arrive at our hotel before sunrise. But it was a close call.

At that point, we had a couple of hours break before the conference breakfast and opening ceremonies were to commence at 8:30 a.m. Then came the very first speaker that Monday morning, delivering the Keynote presentation. I'm so proud to say that it was Karl, who gave an impressive talk on "New financial risk ratios and portfolio growth angles." Despite the preceding adventures and lack of sleep, he did so without missing a beat. Meanwhile I, despite often sitting in a coma in the audience, managed to attend the rest of the day's events.

Almost a year later, on April 11, 2016, Karl wrote to tell me that he had suffered "a deep-brain hemorrhage" in February that he was in the process of recovering from. "After a week of terrible headaches, finally I 'went down' but somehow still managed to call the Emergency Ambulance service at 4:48 a.m.... Mentally I am fine, although I am not perfect! Also physically. Very lucky! But not teaching."

He would not be attending any conferences soon either, he added.

> Main point: I was invited speaker in Sweden for a Quantum conference, and was considering on same trip to come to one of your three conferences, probably the one for Jeff (Hunter), but have now decided it is too early and I will not be up to speed so: I will come to NO conferences this summer!

Only recently, Karl reminded me in another email, "Little did we all know that [SFTFS-2015] would be my last conference. If you look at my C.V., on page 35 you will find no more conferences listed!"

But let's go back a bit. My first communication with Karl took place in 2000 when I was handling his paper for the *Linear Algebra and its Applications* (LAA), which came to print in 2002. This was the Ninth Special Issue of LAA on Linear Algebra and Statistics. So, if you don't know, I'm a statistician, visiting sometimes as a guest editor in math journal special issues. Karl is mastering one particular topic that I have been interested in for a long time: antieigenvalues. They are related to the efficiency of ordinary least-squares, on which I did my Ph.D. thesis.

The first time I met Karl was at the Tampere Bus Station, on Saturday, June 8, 2002. He had taken a bus from the Helsinki Airport, and so on Sunday, June 9, 2002, my wife Soile and I met Karl around noon in downtown Tampere. We walked along the banks of the rapids of Tammerkoski, a Finnish national landscape. Discussing things to do in Tampere, I mentioned that they were showing *A Beautiful Mind*, a movie about the famous mathematician John Nash. This led to Karl telling us colorful episodes about his communications with John Nash in the 1960s. After a long sunny walk, we drove to our home in Nokia, 20 km away. On the way, we stopped at Kotipizza to fetch a late lunch to be enjoyed on the deck of our sauna.

Since 2002, I have met Karl at conferences in various parts of the world, including in Auckland, New Zealand, in 2005. He always travels with hand luggage only! I easily could go on with my reminiscences about our meetings, but to complete this Foreword to Karl's book *Reverberations of a Stroke* I must not linger. However, just one more note: When I first learned of Karl's stroke in 2016, I immediately responded: "Quite something, Karl! Something to put into your Memoirs, Part II!" Little did I know then that Karl had already begun his writing efforts toward what would become this book.

Having now read the completed manuscript, I can't tell you how pleased and honored I feel to be writing this Foreword. Karl's story already is a great success in my own view.

Karl's account begins on January 31, 2016: "I was aware that something unusual was happening to me, although I was not sure exactly what." He then describes, deeply, how the stroke and subsequent emergency medical procedures on 1 February, 2016, drastically changed his life: "From the moment I became aware, while still in the hospital, that 'stroke' was the condition I'd endured and death was what I'd narrowly escaped, I became determined to defeat both conditions."

Karl's description of getting a second life (as he puts it) makes for sharp and touching reading. And there is a determination in Karl that creates a sense of great positivity and inspiration for the reader. I would not be surprised to see Karl's book resting on bedside tables in stroke rehab centers around the world.

Simo Puntanen
Faculty of Natural Sciences
University of Tampere
Tampere, Finland

# Foreword by Jillian Lloyd: *Going to See Karl*

As I walked down the long, echoing hall of the former Boulder Community Hospital, now housing only its rehabilitation program, the building seemed abandoned. Except for a security guard at the front desk, who directed me down the cavernous hall to an elevator, I saw no one and heard only my own footsteps. I felt tense and uncertain of what to expect.

It was February 19, 2016, and Karl had been hospitalized since February 1, when he'd been taken by ambulance to Swedish Medical Center in Denver. I was still fuzzy on details, but I knew he'd suffered a brain hemorrhage, determined to be because of an "arteriovenous malformation" (AVM). I'd never heard of an AVM before, and it meant almost nothing to me; but I knew its implications were dead serious.

I also knew that Karl was recovering well. But no one knew whether he would recover all of his faculties—or if so, when. Karl's friend Kent had emailed to let me know that with Karl now out of Intensive Care, visitors were allowed and encouraged. Kent had also cautioned that Karl might not recognize me and might not be lucid. He had explained that, although conscious and communicative, Karl was still confused and disoriented. Reportedly, Karl kept a notepad by his bedside, which he would refer to when someone entered his room. Kent noticed that Karl had written down a few basic details, including: "My name is Karl Gustafson," "I am a professor of mathematics at the University of Colorado," "I am at Swedish Hospital in Denver."

Without a written note including my name, would Karl recognize me? I worried that he might look blankly at me. I also had no idea of his physical condition. In a sense, would I easily recognize him?

Karl and I have known each other for over a decade, and for as long as I can remember, there has been a wordless understanding between us. We can finish each other's thoughts and sentences and even anticipate them. For this reason, we have always had a wonderful working relationship; but more than that, we are simpatico. As in most situations of connection to others, we assume things will never change. But unwelcome change had come.

When I reached the end of the hall, I found the stairs and mounted to the building's fourth floor. The rehab unit lobby was bright and welcoming, and approaching the nurses' station, the human vibe felt the same. A smiling nurse asked how she could help and if I was there to see someone? She looked searchingly into my eyes, trying to gauge my emotional state, perhaps. She must do this all day long, I thought, try to read and attend to all manner of inner states of concern, distress, and generally blindsided family members and friends. I replied that I had come to see Karl Gustafson. "Room 440," she replied with a smile, sweeping her arm toward the hall. "You can go right in."

Carrying a vase of brightly colored roses, I walked the few steps to Karl's room and entered the open door trying to steel myself for—anything. Karl's bed was faced away from the door, toward a large window and a majestic mountain view. The moment I stepped into the room, Karl turned around and immediately lit up with an enormous grin, his eyes glittering. I breathed a sigh of relief, inwardly, and setting down the flowers, came over to hug him. He hugged back hard. Other than being in a hospital bed, Karl looked almost exactly as when I'd last seen him, on January 29, at the University of Colorado. His color was good, and there were no tubes or wires, not even an IV line. He was sitting partly upright, the head of his bed inclined 45 degrees, with pillows propped behind him. He was wearing a blue button-down shirt—one of his own—rather than hospital garb. He appeared a bit tired, but who wouldn't in such a circumstance? Most of all, he appeared sharp and alert.

There might have been some wishful thinking on my part. I still didn't know if he knew my name or who I was, despite his apparent pleasure at my visit. He studied the roses and commented on how beautiful they were and thanked me for bringing them. Then, he said, "You should put some more water in that vase. Roses need a lot of water." This is true and it gave me a feeling of further relief—that he noticed such a thing. I went to the bathroom sink and topped up the water in the vase. "That's better," he said, when I set the flowers down again.

Then, Karl launched in with great animation: "Do you know what happened to me?" he asked. "Not exactly," I replied honestly. He pointed to the center of the top of his head: "I have a hole here! There's a hole into my brain!" He was referring to the hole that had been drilled for the blood drain. "I don't understand it at all, I don't know how it happened," he went on. "They say I had a brain injury and I don't remember anything. I just remember calling the ambulance, calling 911, early that morning on February 1. But I don't know what happened to me. It all happened so fast. I almost died! I'm lucky to be alive!" He spoke clearly, but chose his words carefully. I nodded, "Yes, you're very lucky."

"I'd had this terrible headache and then I knew something was happening to me," he continued. "It felt like all the energy was draining out of me, and I then heard a voice in my head, telling me, 'Make the call. You must call 9-1-1.' So I did."

"Do you remember anything else before you called 911?" I asked. "Do you remember what you were doing that day?" I was still trying to piece it all together, this non sequitur of seeing Karl hale and seemingly invincible one day, and then learning soon after that he'd suffered a "catastrophic" brain injury.

"I was working on a problem, I'd been working on it for days, and I just couldn't figure it out!" he replied. "I was at my limit, I couldn't do it anymore and I needed help. So I got on the phone, I put in that call to 911 and told them, 'Look, I'm working on this problem and I can't do it alone. You need to send someone over to help me!' And it worked: they sent the ambulance right over. And that saved my life!" He seemed to ponder this miracle, while I tried to sort out whether he'd spoken to the 911 operator about mathematics or strictly about physical symptoms. (The 911 recording would reveal later that there was no mention of math!)

Karl then asked if I could get him some water. He complained that the nurses wouldn't let him have liquids and he was extremely thirsty. I said I'd ask the nurse. She explained that they were restricting Karl's fluids because his sodium levels were low. However, she offered Karl a small ice pop to suck on. He accepted with disappointment, complaining that the nurses were so "strident" about their rules. "They refuse to budge!"

I nodded and mentioned how I remember my young son having to settle for an ice pop, grudgingly, after his surgery a few years ago. Karl perked up and said, "I remember when he had that surgery!" I could tell that he did remember. That was encouraging.

Karl then told me about his visitors: Amy, Garth, Kent, and John had come the day before and would return later. He continued listing visitors who had come and taken walks with him, or joined him for lunch or dinner, and I understood that this was probably imagined or dreamed. One of the friends he mentioned was no longer alive, and another lived in Greece! It was a beautiful late-winter Colorado day, sunny and above 60 degrees. I commented on it and the spectacular view from his window. "Yes!" he said enthusiastically. "We could be in Switzerland! Look at those mountains!" Suddenly he added: "Let's go out for a walk!" He meant right now.

"Yes, we should do that Karl," I replied. "When you feel well enough." I was not sure if he was even allowed to get out of bed without a walker (he wasn't), but his enthusiasm was infectious.

Karl mentioned some issues with short-term memory loss and confusion. "Well, you just have to be patient, Karl, you'll get better. But it might take a while," I observed. I wasn't attempting to placate him; I felt deeply that he would recover. He was silent for a moment and then agreed that he needed to let the process unfold. "There's no hurry, there isn't any place else I need to be," he joked.

Although it's difficult to explain, some of the conversation I had with Karl that day was unspoken—exchanged not in words but with something clearer than that, and I won't attempt to translate it. Urging Karl to take a nap, I hugged and kissed him good-bye and promised to return soon.

Within weeks, Karl had recovered sufficiently to return to his Boulder home. Amazing everyone, he returned to workouts at the gym just a couple of weeks later. As anyone who knows Karl can attest, he is a veritable force of nature, and a stroke—even a catastrophic one—is hardly a match for his determination.

That April, when Karl first mentioned his idea of writing a book about his stroke experience, I was surprised by his confident ambition, but I encouraged him. At the very least, I thought a journaling approach to recording his memories and recovery would be good cognitive and emotional therapy. And I know how much he loves to write, so why not? I really had no idea that he would throw himself into the task with such vigor and enthusiasm; but this is simply how Karl approaches life. As the post-stroke months rolled by, Karl produced chapter after chapter with increasing ease, the steadiness of his cognitive recovery apparent in his written efforts. Now, two years later, he has completed the manuscript of the book before you, a poignant story of one man's struggle to regain his inner balance and life purpose in the aftermath of a near-death health event.

Regardless of the challenges that life throws at Karl, and there have been many, he always seems to land on his feet. What is it that makes some mortals seem so indomitable? I look no further than to Karl and his life for answers. I continue to be inspired by his achievements and have no doubt there will be many more.

Jillian Lloyd
Boulder, CO, USA
April, 2018

# Acknowledgements

There are far too many acknowledgments that I gratefully feel and wish to share; but in the interests of practicality and efficiency, here are a few.

First, to the 911 operator and all of the emergency and medical staff who saved my life and helped in my recovery: Everyone did the right thing. I offer you my humble thanks and permanent gratitude.

Second, to my son Garth who rushed to the emergency room at 7 a.m. to replace the chaplain at my bedside and who then took the entire week off from work to remain by my side daily in the intensive care unit. And equally to my daughter Amy, who flew in from California and who also had the presence of mind to immediately call my department chairman to inform him that I would not be teaching class that week or any time soon.

Third, to all my good and true friends who visited me during my five weeks of hospitalization: Kent Goodrich and John Tracy, who came to Denver often and took the lead in keeping everyone else informed; Norm Nesbit, Mircea Fotino, Doris Goodrich, Bob Leben, Ed McConkey, Al Lundell, Jillian Lloyd—who brought flowers—and Kathy Weakland.

Fourth, to my granddaughters Ashley (16) and Elizabeth (13) who came to the Boulder rehab hospital to cheer me up. I could not remember Elizabeth's name, and I still remember her surprised expression when I had to ask her and then wrote down her reply on a notepad beside me. And also, to my other grandchildren, Francesca (14), Clarissa (11), Julian (11), who came from California to visit me during my recovery.

Fifth, to Donna, who took charge of the paperwork at the Mathematics Department and whose cheerful disposition has kept the department afloat for these many years.

Sixth, and not least, to Jillian Lloyd, who has held my hand and continually encouraged and helped me write this account, while it is still reasonably within my memory's grasp.

Seventh: to this wonderful Encore: A second and more appreciative life!

Karl Gustafson
Boulder, Co, USA
2018

# Contents

# The End

## ...a cold, gray, winter day

1

I awoke on Jan. 31, 2016, to the dawn of a cold, gray, winter day. A heavy snowfall was expected later that day, and I could feel its impending arrival. Groggily, I found my way to my kitchen in search of strong coffee and sustenance. My head ached. I hadn't slept well over the weekend, consumed by a physics problem that had kept me up late and disturbed my dreams, as I turned over and over in my mind the possible solutions, without feeling any nearer to the breakthrough I needed. But I wasn't giving up.

For now, however, I just needed to get rid of this unmerciful headache.

The headache had been going on for several days already, and it seemed to be an after-effect of a flu I'd contracted the week before. I don't normally get bad headaches, but this one wouldn't quit. Was I under too much stress? Was I working too hard? I had just returned a few weeks before to teaching at the University of Colorado after a one-year sabbatical. Of course, I'd worked hard during that sabbatical year too—delivering four keynote speeches around the world! But returning back to the grind of Math Department politics and daily demands was an adjustment; and I was 80 years old, after all. Most of my contemporaries had long since retired.

After a bowl of cold cereal and a steaming cup of coffee, I sat down to my usual routine of reading the Sunday newspaper. In the back of my mind I knew I should start working on the presentation I would give in Växjo, Sweden, where I'd been invited to speak at a Quantum Mechanics conference in late June, 2016. I have this deep problem in physics that I wanted to expose there, and I've been thinking on it for years. I just needed to work up a draft.

After a while, I put the newspaper aside, but still I could not bring myself to tackle the Sweden talk. Then I thought, "You should take a walk". It was cold out—well below freezing—but I put on my down parka and out I went to do my usual 15-minute loop in the bracing fresh winter air. The sky was overcast, but I could still clearly see the softened outline of the towering mountains to the west, and the frost of my breath with each exhale. It felt good to be out walking, so I extended the route to a 30-minute loop.

© Springer Nature Switzerland AG 2019
K. Gustafson, *Reverberations of a Stroke*,
https://doi.org/10.1007/978-3-030-12862-3_1

When I got back home, it was already afternoon. Then I showered and shaved and sat down to a simple lunch of a turkey sandwich and glass of orange juice. Afterwards, I would certainly climb the stairs to my second-floor office and get to work on the Sweden talk; that was my definite plan. But then I felt unusually tired, and my headache remained, so instead I went to my bedroom and took a nap, falling into a deep, dreamless sleep.

By the time I awoke, it was already dark, well after 5 p.m. As I tried to clear my head and raise some energy, I opened and heated a can of tomato soup and served myself a large bowl. Then I decided I needed to be more awake before getting down to work. Lately I had gotten into the habit of watching "60 Minutes" on television at 6 p.m., and I did so. I continued to avoid the pressure of drafting the Sweden talk and then watched an episode of the French murder mystery "Maigret" on television (Channel 252, "programming for a globally minded audience"). It must have been 9 p.m. when it concluded, and at that point I decided I was too wiped out to do anything constructive. And my head still ached. I simply could not go upstairs and think about the Sweden talk.

I truly wanted to go to the conference in Sweden, I love Sweden. But I knew I couldn't yet answer the question I planned to raise in the talk there. That was the obstacle I faced and I could not see a way around it. So I picked up a magazine and read until I was ready to retire to bed.

That night, however, I could not sleep. The headache had not abated at all, and without any activities to preoccupy me and distract my mind, the heavy persistent pain kept me awake. I also felt guilty about not working on the Sweden talk. With both stresses weighing on me, I got up, jotted down a few notes, and poured myself a glass of milk—using it to down an aspirin.

The next thing I remember is that I was sitting on my living room sofa with some notepads scattered around me. I was aware that something unusual was happening to me, although I was not sure exactly what. I wrote out a note to my housecleaning couple apologizing for having the flu. "Hi Sally and Jack" I wrote in a page-long letter to them in neat cursive, describing my "extreme tiredness" and having a headache so bad that "I felt like dying at one point!".

Instinctively I knew then that I wouldn't be home in the morning when they arrived, or that I wouldn't be at my regular yoga class at noon, or teaching my Partial Differential Equations class at the University that afternoon. I pulled out my daypack and placed a few necessary items inside: my pajamas, toilet kit, and a change of underwear and socks. On the coffee table, I left out a Durable Power of Attorney document for my son Garth.

Suddenly, I began to feel the energy draining out of me as if somebody had pulled a plug. Then I heard a forceful voice inside me, urging firmly: "Make the call, fella. You MUST make the call." All parts of my mind that were not paralyzed by pain must have come together to warn me that I was going down fast. I sat there with my iPhone in my hands, looked at it intently, and then managed to tap out 9–1–1 (for the first time in my life). It was 4:48 a.m. on the morning of Feb. 1, 2016.

I don't remember anything about that call now, but out of curiosity I recently obtained a copy of the 911 recording. My voice sounded noticeably weak and fatigued as I told the 911 operator that I'd been "fighting a flu" for 10 days, along with "terrible headaches". Then I stated emphatically: "I absolutely need an ambulance to go to an emergency room." The operator reassured me soothingly that help was being dispatched right away. As he continued to query me about my symptoms, I described "intolerable pain" in my head, neck, and spine, which "had gotten much worse tonight". The call lasted 3 minutes. Then I waited for the ambulance. At the bottom of the note to Sally and Jack, I scrawled in a shaky hand: "CORRECTION called 911 at 4 a.m.,"… but I did not finish the sentence. That's the last thing I remember.

\* \* \*

It had begun to snow heavily early on Feb. 1, and over a foot of snow would fall on Boulder before the end of the day, although I recall nothing of it. I would learn from Garth much later that, when the ambulance arrived at 4:58 a.m., the paramedics found me pacing in my living room, wearing my little daypack.

# Twilight and Dawn

**2**

## …a new beginning

I do not remember the ambulance ride nor its drivers who came quickly to pick me up after my 911 call early on Feb. 1. I remember nothing of the 20-mile drive to Exempla Good Samaritan Hospital in the nearby town of Lafayette. I have no mental image of any of the medical personnel who worked to save my life in the Emergency Room. Indeed, from the time that I placed the 911 call until nearly three weeks later, I remember almost nothing at all.

I wonder where I was during that time when I'd lost my senses, my mind, my very self. That remains a mystery to me still.

As I pored over my ER medical records for clues, I was surprised to find that initially I'd been admitted as a patient with "altered mental status". What? But it was true that within minutes of making the 911 call at 4:48 a.m., I'd lost my mental faculties. The ambulance drivers reported that when they had arrived, a mere 10 minutes later, I could not remember why I had called them.

The Exempla Hospital emergency room admission report states that I appeared younger than my stated age and was initially conscious and alert, but "pleasantly confused". I could not tell them why I was there. I reported that I'd been there the previous day, which was quickly determined to be untrue. My condition then deteriorated rapidly, and I became comatose with the onset of respiratory failure as cerebral bleeding spread into the surrounding tissues of my brain.

A breathing tube was placed quickly and a stroke alert called. Via a CAT scan and CT angiogram, the doctors determined that an arteriovenous malformation (AVM) at the base of the third ventricle had burst, with blood hemorrhaging into all four ventricles of my brain. The AVM was considered too deep and too dangerous to be operable. Instead, the doctors performed an emergency "ventriculostomy"—a surgical procedure that involves drilling a hole into the skull and placing a drain tube into the brain.

Essentially, an AVM is a "tangle" of blood vessels in the brain, and it's typically a congenital condition. Presumably I had lived all of my 80 years with this ticking time bomb inside my brain.

© Springer Nature Switzerland AG 2019
K. Gustafson, *Reverberations of a Stroke*,
https://doi.org/10.1007/978-3-030-12862-3_2

When my son Garth arrived at the hospital at 7 a.m., he was met first by the hospital chaplain. The situation was dire—what my doctor later described as a "catastrophic bleed". I was in critical condition and given a 50–50 chance of survival. The hospital advised Garth to go to my house and see if he could locate any papers that would indicate my medical wishes.

Given the complexities of my condition, I was to be transferred immediately by helicopter to Swedish Medical Center Hospital in Denver, which has a comprehensive Stroke Center. But the blizzard intervened and all helicopters were grounded; instead I was transported by ambulance. I would remain in the Critical Care Unit at Swedish Hospital for the next two weeks.

My next memory came on Feb. 3, two days later, when Garth asked me to sign my name, authorizing some procedure. I remember struggling to do so, but finally managing it. Garth says it took me three attempts to sign my name, and then I wanted to keep signing it! By then, I was recovering well from the "blood drain" procedure, talking and even able to stand up (with help). The doctors said I was dramatically exceeding expectations for a person of my age with my condition.

I have no other memories of my stay at Swedish Hospital, but I know that I was transferred out of Critical Care only for my last two days there, and that Garth came daily during that first week to be at my side. Evidently I did not want to eat anything for most of that period and lost about 15 lb. From Garth I also learned that the neurosurgeon Dr. Adam Hebb at Swedish decided right away that the AVM and ruptured aneurism were too deep for surgery, and therefore it was necessary to wait for the blood to stop draining and hope for the best.

My daughter Amy in California meanwhile conferred with doctors and Garth, charting the course of my treatment. Apparently within a few days I was much improved, to the great relief of my family and friends, who had been preparing for the worst.

The hospital reports indicated that I tolerated all procedures well. But as far as I can tell, my senses were turned off during that time and I did not even experience pain. In fact, it was not until weeks later that I realized that my right arm was partially paralyzed.

On Feb. 17, I was moved to a rehab center at Boulder Community Hospital. Although still in a fog when I arrived there, my mind did turn on briefly as I entered a brightly lit and seemingly friendly room, which looked like a hotel lobby. I was asked to sign something. This turned out to be at the admissions desk on the fourth floor of the old Boulder Community Hospital building, which had been converted to an inpatient rehabilitation unit. I would remain there for the next 20 days.

Upon arrival, I felt a tangible happiness. This may have been my first distinctly felt emotion since the occurrence of the stroke. I cannot say why exactly. Maybe it was because I was back in Boulder, even though I did not consciously know it then. But did a sixth sense somehow know? I am not sure that I would have ever recovered if I had remained in Denver. I have always loved Boulder and prefer to avoid Denver.

Now back in Boulder, I gradually found my way out of a rather profound confusion. I began to recognize faces and my surroundings. My vision, which had been badly blurred until that point, began to clear up. My hearing, however, remained damaged: the words were, and still are, hard to separate.

# Going Home

**3**

## ...negotiating rehab and reality

Back in Boulder, I settled comfortably into a small private room in the rehab unit, with a window framing an uplifting view of the mountains beyond. Within a few days, my mental awareness was returning and I had a better understanding of my medical situation. I remember particularly having the clear conscious feeling of a joy of life. I was alive! A second life beckoned me.

I also remember becoming cognizant that my room was in the same hospital where I'd had knee surgery twice before, at ages 20 and 40. It occurred to me that I might be in the same room where I'd recovered from my knee surgery in 1975. That thought brought me comfort and somehow seemed to bode well. From my hospital bed I gazed out my window at the familiar scenery of home. Something about that beautiful landscape and of what lay beyond the walls of the hospital building supplied me with an inner resolve. I was palpably aware of how much I wanted to recover and walk out of the doors of that hospital—sooner rather than later. That feeling carried me along.

A few days later, as I lay in bed one morning feeling exhausted, I became aware of my own mind prompting me: "It is up to you, Karl! If you do not get up from this bed, you will be here forever." That was how my mind intuitively understood my prospects. I remember that moment distinctly, and how I consciously harnessed all my mental resources and will and determined that I *would* get up.

Months later I would have a discussion with a famed brain injury specialist who has spent a lot of time in hospital wards. He told me that it's always a mystery who decides to get up and who essentially gives up: It really is up to the patient and there's only so much that doctors and medical staff can do. Personality may have much to do with it, I suppose, and it's not in my nature to give up. It never has been.

Friends and family could more easily visit me now that I was in the acute rehab unit. I had a lot of visitors and I'm sure that their caring support played an enormous role in my rapid recovery. I was not always lucid for visitors, however. When my son Garth brought my two granddaughters, ages 11 and 14, to visit for the first time, I still remember looking at Elizabeth, the younger child, and asking, "What is your name?" It had slipped away from me. Eyes wide, she did not answer at first, wondering if I might be joking. When she finally responded, "Elizabeth," I was able

© Springer Nature Switzerland AG 2019
K. Gustafson, *Reverberations of a Stroke*,
https://doi.org/10.1007/978-3-030-12862-3_3

to restore the lost connections. "And that would be your sister Ashley over there," I replied, gesturing to my eldest grandchild. This is an example of the extreme value of a clue, or just some association, in how neural networks function. It recalls to me the ground-breaking research of Yaser Abu-Mostafa on artificial intelligence in the late 1980s, when I was involved in that field.

Another day early on, I remember my friends Ed, Bob, John, Kent, Kathy, Norm, Mercia, and Jillian all visiting me at once. I remember wondering whether they didn't mind being crowded into the small room together. But of course they were not all there at once! My temporal lobe time scales were still out of whack and my mind had somehow compressed their visits, probably over a period of days, into one visit.

Jillian had brought me some flowers when she visited during that first week. But when I admired them on my bedside table later that day, I had no idea where they had come from. I had to ask the nurse: "Did someone bring me these flowers?"

At that point, my short-term memory was seriously deficient, whereas my long-term memory seemed mostly intact. Whether and when my short-term memory would begin to function properly was unknown; but for now, it was a real problem. A nurse or therapist would introduce herself, and five minutes later I could not recall her name. Or in the midst of a conversation with a visiting friend, I might forget what we were talking about. I suppose I repeated myself a lot.

My daughter Amy flew in from California for several days and she and Garth were told to come up with a Plan B in the event that I could not return home. No one had any idea at that time whether I would be able to live independently again. But I don't think I ever doubted it.

A night nurse had to wake me often to take a blood sample. One concern was that I was suffering from a condition called hyponatremia, in which the body won't maintain adequate sodium levels. This apparently was a consequence of the stroke and cerebral bleeding. The condition worsened my symptoms of mental confusion and tiredness, since the brain needs the proper balance of sodium and potassium in order for the synapses to function properly. To combat this, I was required to take salt tablets, and my fluid intake was very restricted until my sodium levels came up and finally stabilized. But still I had to continue taking the salt tablets.

The young floor doctor was named Dr. Tsoi. She called me Professor Gustafson rather than "Karl", which I liked very much. It helped remind me of my old self and further motivated me to recover.

After a week I was moved to a grandiose room occupying the entire southwest corner of the fourth floor. It was called "the penthouse" and its large windows on two sides of the room provided striking views of the mountains. A plaque on the wall indicated that the room had been donated by a Professor Richard McCray and his wife Sandra. Professor McCray was now retired from the Astrophysics Department at the University, but I vividly recalled having locked horns with him in the past at Arts & Sciences faculty meetings. Now I put the past aside and thanked him in low tones for my fine penthouse. Perhaps this was the first episode post-stroke in which I was evolving into a new mind-frame: Forget the small stuff and get out of the blame game.

Each day, I had three or four hour-long rehab sessions. A collateral motivation was to get you up and moving. It was the same for meals: You were expected to eat your meals in the dining room with the other patients. Each morning, while we were still in bed, we patients would be given a printed schedule of the day's sessions. You needed to get yourself up and to the appointed locations at the appointed times, using your wheelchair, walker, or cane as necessary. This could be surprisingly difficult to accomplish when, at times, I just wanted to stay in bed and sleep. Then when I would rouse myself, I often had difficulty remembering the locations of the various therapy rooms, including for Speech, Physical, and Occupational therapy.

All the therapists were female and I liked them all. One I recall was a hard-ass, partly by design, and I suspect partly by personality. But I accepted that. Soon I surmised that I would not be going home until each of them could sign off on my readiness. This motivated me to work as hard as I could.

I never figured out exactly what the different therapy sessions were aiming to accomplish. But I knew that I had to accomplish those goals, whatever they were. Of course I knew Physical Therapy was to restore one's physical movement. Fortunately, I moved well and by chance I had not been paralyzed by the stroke. I had only some partial paralysis in my right hand. But I was on my feet and could walk a straight line.

Occupational Therapy was less well defined. It seemed to mean being able to return to work, whether that work was at home, an office, or in laying bricks.

Speech Therapy was the humdinger! A better name might be: Brain Therapy. Sometimes I had two sessions per day. I had to pass examinations on my hearing, sight, and various cognition tasks. Initially I was quite slow on some of the cognitive endeavors. Looking back, I now realize that these were Left Brain tasks, and my Left Brain was damaged. But I stuck to it and prevailed.

Only briefly did I use a walker to make my way through the halls. But I must laugh now at my attachment to a walking stick that the physical therapist, Lisa, had supplied to me. It was made of wood, perfectly straight, and more than an inch in diameter, with a wide rubber base. I took it everywhere with me, to meals, to therapy sessions, and even to the bathroom. I soon convinced Lisa that I was ready to go outside and we would take half-hour walks in the nearby neighborhood with my wondrous walking stick. Quickly I began to scheme how I could talk someone into letting me take the walking stick home. The staff seemed to humor me; no one said yes and no one said no. Somehow the walking stick had become my personal security blanket and I did not want to give it up.

I have since seen identical walking sticks at the local hardware store. Luckily, I have no further need for one. I am convinced that being able to walk freely is a great rehabilitation accelerator, especially as compared to being confined to a wheelchair.

I enjoyed eating my meals at a small table in the dining room with my new friends Helen and Harry, who were also recovering from strokes. Helen was about my age and widowed. She still needed a walker to get around. Harry was mentally sharp and possessed a sly sense of humor, and he was physically robust despite a misshapen arm from childhood polio. Both were, I would say, good company and good for the soul. It's important to be surrounded by positive forces and influences during challenging times. Generally I have not been overly sympathetic to the claims of the Social Sciences, but this experience convinced me that when it comes to our minds, the effects of human interactions are fundamental.

I remember a pretty therapist named Fara. She was petite and wore blue jeans and told me that she was of Middle-Eastern extraction. I imagined Persian. We had chemistry, or at least I felt chemistry. I thought I heard her say one day that she loved me. Did I imagine that? On being required to buy, prepare, and cook a meal to demonstrate my competence for returning home, she volunteered to take me to the market across the street and then be my lunch guest. I chose to make us a favorite meal of spinach salad and omelets, which was a great success.

I wondered if some of my male friends who have never cooked could pass such an "exam". Maybe they waive the test for men who are returning home to their wives. Too bad for them! I have always found my time in the kitchen to be good general therapy.

Eventually it became clear that I was doing well and could be considered a candidate for going home. One day I and all my therapists met with the rehab director and my son Garth in the small council room. My daughter Amy connected via Skype from California. Each therapist gave a report on me, which indicated my readiness for going home. But the hard-ass speech therapist had reservations. My hearing loss seemed considerable, she said, and she had noticed at times that I was unpredictably impulsive. She also recommended that if I were to go home, I should learn meditation. At this remark, I spoke up: I already attended a weekly meditation class (and have for years) and I would continue to do that. I agreed with her other comments, but countered that I had lived for 47 years in my home, raising a family there as well as living on my own for many years. I could handle it, I said.

The director proposed a compromise: Would I pay for a 24-hour home care service for the first three days home? If all went well, then I could continue on my own thereafter. I agreed enthusiastically. All agreed. And then on Mar. 8, I returned home. It was just over a month since my unplanned departure via ambulance on Feb. 1. And what a glorious day it was! I have never been happier to be back at home.

# The Brain

# 4

## ...mind and meaning

I did not really need them, but the caregivers of Home Care of the Rockies were all very nice. After the mandatory 72 hours of round-the-clock home supervision, I was finally home alone. I slept a lot: the sleep of deep exhaustion, recovering from all those weeks of the hospital protocol of waking the patient constantly. I really needed some rest. I also enjoyed my own kitchen, roaming around the house, looking at the mountains, taking short walks in the neighborhood, and buying groceries at the nearby supermarket. I have been my own "caretaker" since my wife Rose died in 1980—long ago—so this was a familiar lifestyle to me.

I still had to complete a couple of Outpatient Rehab classes before regaining my certification to drive. Two weeks later, my outpatient occupational therapist Karen gave me essentially a driver's license exam. I passed! On Mar. 22, I was mobile again and free as a bird. I didn't really drive far, but now I was able to meet my retired colleagues for workouts at the gym and lunches on campus. A week later, I returned to my regular yoga classes, which were recommended as a valuable rehabilitation tool.

Only then did my mind start to ask: what really happened to me? Besides being a mathematician, I am also a physicist and engineer. My trained scientific curiosity, 60 nonstop years of it, was evidently alive and well. I had never hesitated to dive into new scientific domains and I now decided: it is time to research the brain.

I at least had some background from which to draw. I had performed research on neural networks off and on for 30 years. From the mathematical point of view, I knew the Nobel-prize winning Hodgkin-Huxley electrochemical partial differential equations that described individual neural synapses. But now my interest was centered on the physics. What happens in a stroke? I wanted a general answer, but also, some answers pertinent to my own stroke.

Stroke connotes brain and I realized that I did not really know many details about the human brain. All my life I have had the habit of reading voraciously about anything that interests me. And so for weeks on end, I read everything I could get my hands on about the brain. Of course I freely consulted the internet. And I became particularly enthralled with a fine illustrated book, *The Human Brain Book,* by medical writer Rita Carter, et al. (Penguin, 2014). I still display this

© Springer Nature Switzerland AG 2019
K. Gustafson, *Reverberations of a Stroke*,
https://doi.org/10.1007/978-3-030-12862-3_4

volume prominently on my living room coffee table. Also helpful was the renowned book *My Stroke of Insight: A Brain Scientist's Personal Journey,* by neuroanatomist Jill Bolte Taylor (Viking, 2008). By coincidence, Taylor's stroke in 1996 was also an AVM *(arteriovenous malformation),* the relatively rare type of hemorrhagic stroke that I had suffered.

As a scientist, I began forming my own preferred mental models. If you talk to scientists, you soon learn that they all carry their preferred mental pictures. These models need not be completely accurate; scientists understand that their mental images are not the whole truth. Still, they are an extremely helpful aid to intuition. I expect it must be the same with carpenters, plumbers, and other skilled craftsmen.

For example, Taylor includes rough sketches of her models of the brain throughout her book. Carter's book is mostly pictorial illustrations, accompanied by text explanations. On one page an AVM is pictured and described as an abnormal knot of blood vessels that are subject to rupture. Simply put, these congenital tangles, in which the arteries and veins are not sufficiently separated by an intervening capillary system, may burst (or not) during your lifetime.

In Taylor's case, her AVM was on the left side of her brain, near the scalp, and operable. I knew that my own AVM was located in the lower back center of the brain, inoperable, and when it ruptured, it sent blood into all four ventricles. The third ventricle was affected first. Ventricles: what are those? They are generally described as cavities within the brain containing your cerebrospinal fluid. But they are more interesting than that. I call the four brain ventricles the Great Lakes of the brain. There are two above, left and right, a third one in the center, and the fourth ventricle lies below it, in the upper part of the medulla, with the cerebellum forming its roof.

The ventricles manufacture and contain your cerebrospinal fluid and are all connected and also connected to the thin layer of subarachnoid cerebrospinal fluid that surrounds and cushions the brain. Cerebrospinal fluid entering the fourth ventricle exits to the subarachnoid space of the spinal column, moving through two lateral apertures and a single midline aperture. In my own mental picture, like a map of the Great Lakes, the top two ventricles are Lake Superior and Lake Michigan, which feed into the third ventricle Lake Huron, and then flow down the Detroit River into the fourth ventricle lakes of Erie and Ontario and finally to the St. Lawrence Seaway.

My AVM was located at the base of the third ventricle, and according to the hospital ER reports, by the time it was diagnosed it had pulsed blood into all four ventricles and the subarachnoid brain cushion. The AVM measured just $2.1 \times 2.3$ cm, almost a square inch. I like to picture it as covering all of Detroit in the U.S. and Windsor across the river in Canada. One reason this picture appeals to me comes from my visit to Windsor in 2007 to give a lecture at a conference there. I was struck by how beautiful the skyline of Detroit was when seen in the evening from across the river in Windsor. In my "brain model", both cities were wiped out by a massive flood of blood erupting from that river basin.

I theorize that my ten days of severe headaches preceding the stroke were caused by my AVM slowly leaking blood but not yet bursting into my four ventricles.

If so, that early continuously leaking pressure-release may have saved my life. Certainly it warned me that something was seriously wrong, although I did not know what at the time. In retrospect, it's amazing that the idea of a stroke never even entered my mind.

\* \* \*

Having a stroke invariably means that some parts of your brain will die. These parts do not grow back. Instead, other parts of the brain will attempt to take over the lost functions. This mechanism is called brain plasticity, or neuroplasticity. From neuroscientists we know that the brain is enormously plastic at any age, and that brain activity associated with a damaged portion of the brain often can be transferred to a different location. This is an example of positive plasticity, and it tends to occur naturally in the process of recovery from an acute brain injury such as a stroke.

There are two quite different kinds of strokes. Most strokes are *ischemic*: caused by a clot in a brain artery. I call this *a local drought*. Only about 10% are *hemorrhagic*: caused by an artery rupturing somewhere in the brain. I call this *a local flood*. Of the latter type, about one in fifty is a ruptured *AVM*. It seems to me that everybody should be aware of the difference. You do not treat a drought and a flood in the same way! For example, I should never take any blood thinning medication.

In the Emergency Room, they had detected that I was losing feeling on the right side of my body. Your right side is controlled by your Left Brain. By this I mean only, without going into precise detail, that it's governed by parts of the left side of your brain. It was not until week three after the stroke that I was cognizant enough to notice that my right arm and right hand were partially paralyzed. But after performing special exercises for a few weeks, the feeling and control in my right hand and arm gradually returned. I was very lucky.

\* \* \*

Left Brain and Right Brain. This dichotomy, even if not exact, and certainly not complete, is now widely accepted, and has come to fascinate me. A main thread running through Jill Bolte Taylor's book is her coming to better appreciate her Right Brain, even to the extent of deciding to not try to restore some of her Left Brain functions. My own experience has been similar. Living by one's Right Brain seems to be better for one's happiness. And maybe better for the happiness of others.

To the Left Brain are attributed the qualities of logic, analysis, mathematics, thinking in words, and language. To the Right Brain are attributed creativity, intuition, imagination, thinking in images, and facial recognition. The two sides of the brain of course communicate with each other regularly.

Some would simplify even further, claiming that your Left Brain is your ego, and your Right Brain is your soul. I won't go that far, but I will stipulate here that your Left Brain is your *mind* and your Right Brain is your *meaning*. What do I get up for in the morning, why bother to keep living? My Right Brain supplies the answer. Then how do I carry that out, how do I survive? My Left Brain answers.

I have published in the physics community that studies consciousness. They like the words *ontological* and *epistemological*. The first connotes objective reality

(Left Brain) and the second connotes subjective reality (Right Brain). The Left Brain tries to be objective. The Right Brain tries to be subjective.

My university education took me through engineering, business, physics, and then mathematics. I ended up in a pure mathematics department, but I have never been fully comfortable there. They tend to view everything as correct, or wrong: In other words, you can either supply a proof (Left Brain) or you cannot (Right Brain); there is no "in-between". I have come to see this as living in a black-and-white world. And I prefer to live in a Technicolor world.

Politically: Socialism is left-brained, Capitalism is right-brained. Socialism is good theory, Capitalism is good reality. I remember long ago when I arrived in Europe for my first postdoctoral, and a young German physicist at the Battelle Institute in Geneva joked with me: Communism boasted all the equations except for the most important one, the human equation.

Since my stroke I have managed very little mental activity in terms of logic, analysis, and mathematics. The writing of these chapters has not been easy. But it has been creative, intuitive, and imaginative. It has been worth getting up for in the morning. Thanks to the stroke wiping out of parts of my Left Brain, it has been easier for me to take leave of the Mathematics Department and thereby face retirement. I have come to prefer the happiness of my Right Brain.

Exactly why my Right Brain was spared, I don't know. Instead, I find it poetic that my stroke occurred in the center of my brain and yet my Right Brain prevailed, as it has throughout my life, thereby resolving a lifelong struggle between the left and right hemispheres of my brain.

# Gamma Knife

5

## …dissolving tangles

Through a thick snowstorm in late March, my good friend John drove me down to Denver to meet with Dr. Ari Ballonoff at St. Joseph's Hospital. Our mutual friend Kent came along to lend additional moral support and advocacy as needed. Dr. Ballonoff is a radiation oncologist, and although I don't have cancer, a favored treatment for brain AVMs like mine is to deliver a precise, high-concentration dose of radiation directly into the tangle of blood vessels. This is the same way doctors treat certain types of cancers, including brain tumors. The radiosurgery instrument typically used is called a Gamma Knife.

This instrument is not a knife at all, of course. And while technically non-invasive, the treatment is not without risks—we're talking here about zapping radiation into my brain! As a physicist, it did not feel natural to consider volunteering for intense radiation. Still, this was the course of treatment recommended by the consulting neurosurgeons even in the early morning hours of my stroke: If I survived, they said, I should certainly undergo radiosurgery treatment to destroy or at least diffuse the AVM tangle in the center of my brain. It would be a one-time shot, and I would have to wait two years to know if it had worked. If it succeeded, it would mean a significant reduction in the likelihood of my experiencing a future bleed. So here I was to consult with the expert, who would need to approve of and oversee any treatment plan.

"I'm looking for an 80 year-old man!" Dr. Ballonoff exclaimed with a wry smile when he entered the stark hospital exam room where John, Kent, and I sat waiting. "I'm the patient," I said, accepting the compliment on behalf of the three of us, who try to stay in shape. In the course of frank conversation, Dr. Ballonoff revealed that this treatment "is considered optional" for patients over 75. This could be taken to mean that we might die of something else rather soon. (It also may reflect a rationing of the nation's medical costs.) But in my case, the doctor recommended that I proceed with the radiosurgery treatment, noting that I was in excellent overall health and a good candidate. He also reiterated what I had heard before: that my bleed had been "catastrophic" and a second bleed might be fatal. A reasonable chance at being able to prevent a future bleed was worth taking.

© Springer Nature Switzerland AG 2019
K. Gustafson, *Reverberations of a Stroke*,
https://doi.org/10.1007/978-3-030-12862-3_5

As we continued chatting, I asked Dr. Ballonoff if he thought I could still "climb some 14ers", considering my medical situation. Deftly evading the question, he replied that he had climbed all 54 of Colorado's 14,000-foot peaks. I replied, "Me too, many times over in some cases!" A bond was established between us, as fellow mountaineers. The importance of patient-doctor relations once again impressed upon me. Even though my question was left unanswered, I recognize that probably I'm the only one who can answer it. And that may take some time.

I was to return to St. Joseph's for two more appointments, accompanied again by John and Kent, my loyal friends and retired colleagues. During the first appointment, the technicians took precise measurements of my AVM and its location in my brain, pinpointing the exact location where the radiation was to be delivered. The second appointment, on Apr. 18, was for the Gamma Knife procedure itself. This turned out to be a deceptively short and simple affair. Fully clothed, you lay in a supine position on a padded table and a technician places a mask over your face and bolts it into place. Then the Gamma Knife is positioned precisely—here you must put complete faith in the technician—and then focused beams of gamma radiation are blasted directly into the AVM for about 20 minutes. During this time I felt nothing. But as a physicist, I knew that I had been hit with a lot of radiation. More specifically, with gamma rays, which have extremely short wavelengths and are emitted by atomic nuclei. So I got zapped by very high frequency radiation (and higher photon energies). Of course even lower frequency ultraviolet light from the sun can burn you.

Afterwards I felt perfectly normal and was not aware of any side effects. I did sleep a bit fitfully that night, but I'm not sure there was any connection to the treatment, at least physically. Now I must wait two years to find out whether the Gamma Knife was of any benefit to the AVM tangle. On the other hand, if something went wrong, I'm likely to know sooner.

* * *

As the month of April draws to a close, I realize that three full months have passed since the stroke. There was a lot of action in there. Perhaps this is how it feels to survive combat in a wartime campaign. Now it is over. All the action is over.

I have been released from nearly all contact with the medical community. I had agreed to continue seeing a speech therapist once a month as an outpatient. But beyond that, I am on my own. So what now?

# Perchance to Dream

6

## ...a first mathematical thought

I awoke on a Saturday morning, almost seven months after the stroke, via a distinct dream. I did not want to be late for a 10 a.m. memorial service for the son of a colleague. A few days earlier, tragically, he had fallen or jumped from a high place. I had just had lunch with this fine boy and his mother a few weeks ago, when we had spotted each other at a restaurant in our local shopping center. I'd always had a high opinion of my colleague. Indeed, she was one of the few in the department whom I considered to be "glue". And her son, a recent college graduate, was bright and full of promise. I wondered how my colleague and her family would cope with this unthinkable event.

But now I was late. Why had I not heard the alarm go off? I quickly dressed and rushed out to my car, only to find that the key would not work. I thought: I'll use my older car instead. So I rushed back to the house, but then the house key would not fit the lock either. The hands on the clock now read slightly past 10 a.m. Wait, I am not inside my house, I thought. What is that clock?

Then I heard the alarm with its irritating high-pitched buzz. I rolled over in bed to turn it off and became aware that I had not yet arisen. The bedside clock read 8:40 a.m., as it should. To my relief! As I got up and assembled myself for that sad day, it occurred to me that this was the first dream I could actually remember since having the stroke.

Dreams come from your subconscious, it is presumed. Was this a good sign, then, possibly indicating that my conscious and unconscious thoughts were now separating? My life since the stroke had been that of living in a daze. For a long while, there had been no distinct conscious thinking. I got along well enough, I went through the motions. But while my conversations mostly were rational (except during the first few weeks when they would veer off into imagined fantasy after a rational beginning), I had the feeling that I was relying essentially upon instinct as I reconstructed my life. I felt like I was in an auto-pilot mode. Instinct, unconscious, intuition, I cannot pin it down, but essentially there had been no conscious planning or any goals for the day unless I forced myself to write something down. As my brain slowly healed, it had declared to me: Do not stress me yet!

© Springer Nature Switzerland AG 2019
K. Gustafson, *Reverberations of a Stroke*,
https://doi.org/10.1007/978-3-030-12862-3_6

I now maintained two calendars in my kitchen, a large one on the wall and a smaller one beside the telephone, onto which I would record all my commitments and whatever else I needed to remember. Daily I would consult both calendars to ensure that I would appear for any scheduled appointments. My own memory was not sufficiently reliable.

* * *

The memorial service for the boy took place at St. Aidan's Episcopal Church, very close to the University of Colorado campus. That church happened to be built on a plot that had been the location of our family home when my parents had moved us to Boulder in the summer of 1948, direct from Iowa. Our address had been 2432 Pennsylvania Avenue, and our small frame house was then situated on a dirt road heading east out of town. Now the address is 2425 Colorado Avenue and the church occupies both our former lot and another lot to the west. Four lanes of traffic motors past swiftly. So much has changed. But the little irrigation ditch of fresh mountain water, with which I raised strawberries as a boy of 13 that first summer, still flows steadily along. As I entered the church, I could feel instinct and intuition operating at an elevated level. Quietly, I took a seat in an empty pew and waited for the service.

The randomly chosen church pew where I sat, I thought, could be where my bedroom had been in 1948 in that new but cheap and cold two-bedroom house. My mind wandered back to memories of my boyhood, and then I noticed that some colleagues from the department had joined me in the pew and others were nearby. The family members of the deceased boy gave moving eulogies. My subconscious reminded me of how one of my son's best friends had overdosed during his senior year of high school. His mother had requested that his ashes be placed on my land high in the mountains, where the boys had enjoyed so many happy adventures. And then the mother continued on with her life. Her cheerfulness could not be damped. I always admired her for that.

* * *

Today marks seven months and two days since the stroke. This morning, almost a week after the first remembered dream, I awoke to another rather extraordinary event, similarly without warning. It too emerged from that shadow area between sleep and waking.

I had awakened early this morning, at 6 a.m. instead of at my usual 9 or 10 a.m., and after rising tentatively, I ambled outside to retrieve the morning newspaper. Always hoping to break my post-stroke need for 11–12 hours of sleep at night, I briefly considered staying awake. Instead I relented and went back to bed. I fall asleep easily, but this morning, before I managed to drift off completely, a new mathematical thought flashed abruptly and precisely to my conscious attention: I realized that the Kemeny first-entrance time (which explains why one may start at any initial pure state of a Markov process and expect to arrive in the same amount of time at any other pure state) could be compared to the important Girsanov change of measure, which removes "drift" in the theory of Martingale financial hedge-fund investing. This very technical thought was astonishing! It went beyond the new result I had shared and published last year with statistician and mathematician

Jeffrey Hunter, which was a completely new explanation for Kemeny Time. My paper with Jeff was the last I had written before the stroke, and the hedge-fund theory connection provided another novel twist.

I get very excited when I can create new bridges within mathematics, or even better, between mathematics and related fields. Immediately I sat up in bed and forced myself, still in my pajamas, to write a one-page summary of the pertinent facts and what I believed might be the new mathematical result. I was still not clear how much merit my idea might have. But the critical thing and the most exciting thing for me was that *my mind had awakened mathematically.* It was literally my first mathematical thought since the stroke.

Then I promptly fell back asleep until the alarm woke me for my morning appointment at the gym.

Later, during my pre-lunch walk with Kent and John, I recounted the story of my early-morning breakthrough. Kent had volunteered: "Your subconscious mind has been busy working on it, thrashing it around. But you were not aware of that until it came out as a rational formulation this morning."

I do not disagree with this hypothesis, but the mind remains a great mystery. Insight is by nature spontaneous—but it was nonetheless the spontaneity that surprised me. Until this morning, my mind had refused for seven months to tolerate any level of mathematical thought. I could casually read and speculate on some of my favorite questions in theoretical physics. But when I tried "clicking" on the mathematical parts of my brain, I got nothing. Not merely no reaction, but no energy, no enthusiasm at all. You could have put a pistol to my head and told me to do mathematics, and I would not have been able to.

And this morning, just like that, it returned to me in a dramatic burst. Will there be more of these unbidden thoughts to come? I am hopeful.

# Endless Fatigue

7

## …and the holidays loometh

In the aftermath of the stroke, my greatest challenge seems to be this endless quantity of fatigue. It can be overpowering at times. Fatigue resulting from a stroke is recognized as a different species from normal fatigue. It's not just the physical sort you feel after, say, a hard mountain climb, nor the mental weariness you might feel after a long day at work. Post-stroke fatigue is more like a double whammy, hitting you broadside both mentally and physically to produce a bone-tiredness that chases you at every turn and is impossible to escape from, except in brief intervals.

It's also one of the most frustratingly persistent symptoms for many stroke victims. As the brain heals, it requires an enormous amount of energy. Among other things, the brain is rewiring its circuitry, and the mental tasks that were once performed with ease now may require an enormous amount of focus (if they can be accomplished at all). All of this works as a constant drain upon one's energy resources, mentally and physically. Indeed, it's well-established that the brain uses more of the body's energy than any other organ—and that applies when it's in perfect health. Recovering from any type of brain injury ups the ante substantially.

But stroke fatigue shares an important property with everyday fatigue: You can always address it with the antidote of sleep. While sleep might only keep stroke fatigue at bay temporarily, even that must be counted as a win. So much of our experience of life, and of what we can accomplish, depends on our available energy. And our energy level has a very real impact on our emotional state: Feeling low-energy much of the time is just depressing. And depression saps energy even further still. Personally, I can't afford that. A solution that has worked for me is to make sleep a priority.

Prior to my stroke, I was a typical eight-hours-per-night type of person. I had long been envious of those who regularly needed only six hours of sleep. They had two more hours of the day to get things done, and I like to get things done. I also had wished that I was one of those morning people who wake up at dawn, eager to start their day. The lark, as they say. I was naturally more of a night owl, and I often had to force myself to quit in the evenings, just when I was beginning to get inspired and rolling on some project or another. Back then, I'd rather have stayed awake till dawn than rise with the larks.

© Springer Nature Switzerland AG 2019
K. Gustafson, *Reverberations of a Stroke*,
https://doi.org/10.1007/978-3-030-12862-3_7

But time changes many things. And the stroke changed all of my sleep and wake preferences. We stroke victims are in a separate category, as we are beyond simple preferences to matters of need and functionality. I now regularly sleep 12 hours per night, and I try to get to sleep no later than 10 p.m. When I do this, I function best, and I might not even need an afternoon nap. But if I get only 10 hours of sleep, I find myself after lunch pretty desperate for an additional hour or two of sleep, and must soon succumb to it. With post-stroke fatigue, you really cannot delay getting sleep when that feeling hits.

Further, for me to get through the day with a clear head and any chance at productivity, having adequate sleep and rest is imperative. It took me a while to adjust to this, as I was so used to my "old way" of powering myself through energy lows, perhaps with the aid of a caffeinated beverage. But the old ways work no longer and the price is too high to pay. If I try to force my way through fatigue now, my brain refuses to cooperate, and it more or less abandons me. So there is no more "cutting corners" in the sleep department.

Jill Bolte Taylor reports that it was not until seven years after her stroke that she could reduce her extensive sleep needs. And there was nothing she could do to shorten that time-interval.

There is an important lesson here: Accept the realities you cannot change. And, of course, be grateful for sleep. At least one colleague has, with wry smile, commented that he would love to be able to sleep 12 hours a night! One can fight some problems, but others are best resolved by embracing the new reality. So for now, when I'm tired, I sleep. Without guilt or regret.

Sleep is only one part of the fatigue equation. Another is exercise. Every day I make sure to get out and move physically, whether for a brisk long walk, a session at the gym, or the yoga classes I attend three days a week. (Sometimes it's a combination of all of these endeavors.) Keeping active, even when your energy is low, is a way to feel more energetic and vital, so I make that a daily priority.

I was lucky to have survived my stroke with no bodily paralysis. I am also lucky to be 81 years old. And at this stage of my life, I do not *have to* accomplish more on this Earth. But still I would like to. Nobody wants to be carried off the field, never to play again. Especially when we enjoy the game so, isn't there a little more that we can contribute? I'm still in the game, even if all the rules have changed.

Purpose is another important part of the energy equation, I think. We all need to have purpose and meaning in our lives; without it, why get out of bed in the morning? The fall semester at the university is now underway and I am not teaching. That feels odd to me. A quick calculation revealed that because I had accumulated Sick Leave for more than 45 years before my stroke, I now have more than two years to draw upon. I wonder daily if I will ever return to teaching. Even more, I want to get back into hardnosed mathematical and scientific research if ever I can. But that may not happen, I remind myself. So I continue my shuffle into the days ahead. I will do what I can. But surely I will do something useful with the life I have yet before me. Remaining positive is another essential ingredient, I am certain.

\* \* \*

The calendar brings the holidays closer. I should think about those now. Since 1974, I have supplied a cheese fondue dinner for my family on Christmas Eve. That is now 42 years straight! Will I have the energy to pull it off this year? For 42 years, we have all looked forward to it. We have a special fondue recipe with three imported cheeses, including the coveted Vacherin from the Bernese highlands. Miniature potatoes, sweet gherkins, cocktail onions, and sliced apples are assembled, along with a few other choice supplements and some good white wine, and of course enough two-day-old French baguettes cut properly into bite-size chunks for dipping. The details each year are exactly the same. My son and stepson and even the grandchildren help with the preparations. I now mentally look forward to it. And this year there will be no competing work demands. So it seems clear to me: Just get on with it, Karl, just enjoy it this year! Who knows how many more there will be?

So I take whatever energy I have each day and try to build upon it. And as I build a new life now on the foundation of the old one, I keep my eyes up and my gaze ahead.

# One-Year Anniversary

...acceptance

This week marks the one-year anniversary of my stroke. I have continued on this Earth for one more year and now Feb. 1 feels like another birthday to me. I know very well that it could have gone either way on Feb. 1, 2016. Or for that matter at any point thereafter. Following my stroke, I was told that there was a 26% chance of a second bleed within the first year—which "would probably be fatal", according to my radiology physician. So I am just happy to be here now, one year later. I feel very lucky.

Having a stroke, however, really changes things. Or rather, it changes everything. You simply have to make adjustments. And you must accept the changes the stroke has imposed on you, whether you like it or not. I can't say I have especially liked it, as a matter of fact.

In this year since the stroke, I have just wanted to get back to "my old life". I didn't want any of these changes forced upon me. I kept waiting to get back to doing math, to research, to teaching, and to writing papers, and to delivering invited lectures around the world. Why wouldn't I? That had been my life over the past 60 years ... and it has felt like *who I am*: A mathematician, a professor of mathematics, a world-class player in the world of mathematics. And if I am not a mathematician, then *who am I*? What is my purpose? These were difficult questions for me to examine, much less answer. And I wished that I did not have to, that I could just return to my old self as soon as possible.

And yet, there was the relentless need for sleep and daily naps to stave off the fatigue. Even sleep and naps left me fatigued many times. My energy was about one-half of what it had been before the stroke. Maybe less. My left brain refused to go to work. I wondered, why wouldn't it come back to me and cooperate, attacking math and physics problems like it did for all those years? Would it ever come back?

And could I safely return to climbing mountains, as I have for most of my 81 years? Or must I push the hiking boots and poles to the back of my closet forever?

© Springer Nature Switzerland AG 2019
K. Gustafson, *Reverberations of a Stroke*,
https://doi.org/10.1007/978-3-030-12862-3_8

There were no ready answers to my burning questions and no promises for the future. I have learned that recovery from a stroke is nonlinear and uneven. There are days when the full weight of the changes I have endured rips into me and I carry the burden heavily. Other days I feel quite light and free, brimming over with gratitude.

But still, to relinquish the old life—that prospect seems fairly brutal. I worked so hard to create it, diligently and passionately for all those years. Even now, I feel that *no one wants to be nothing.* That is why retirement can create such an identity crisis for people, particularly for career-driven souls like me. The easiest solution is to just keep on working. So I put up a fight, and I played hard at denial.

From the moment I became aware, while still in the hospital, that "stroke" was the condition I'd endured and death was what I'd narrowly escaped, I became determined to defeat both conditions. Getting out of the rehab was the first step, then returning to living independently again, which I did rather promptly. I surprised everyone by returning to driving within two months of the stroke, along with regularly working out at the gym and attending yoga classes. Without a doubt, I was quickly and diligently putting back together all the pieces of my old life, like rebuilding a smashed-up jigsaw puzzle. Surely the pieces of teaching and math and summiting Colorado's highest mountain peaks would come back into place soon.

I have always been determined. Some would say stubborn. Anyone can tell you that determination, and stubbornness even, are essential ingredients for resilience and recovery from major life catastrophes. So much is about putting one stoic foot in front of the other. That is the approach that has served me well throughout my life, through the myriad challenges and everything else. And for my recovery, I believe this trait of mine was an absolutely essential ingredient. But what I didn't understand until quite recently was that I needed closure to my old life. I needed to find a way toward peace with the loss (death really) of my old life, and to move ahead in the sometimes quite painful transition to the new.

Few of us really like change or embrace it with all our heart. It is just human nature I suppose to want things, especially comfortable things, to stay the same. So how does one muster the courage and ambition to fling open their doors to an unknown new world, filled with new challenges and unknown realities?

In my case, acceptance came only in increments. But there was a crucial turning point a few months ago when I went to consult a neurologist about my prospects and any limitations I might and should expect. I had already asked my personal physician and various rehab workers for plain answers, but when answers came at all they were always vague. While I understood the evasion from their point of view, I decided to press the issue further with the neurologist. As I sat in his office, I had the feeling he already knew what I was up to. So I opened the conversation with a distraction:

Me: "Kurtz. Is that name Austrian or German?"

Dr. Kurtz: "My parents came here from Poland."

Me: "You know, 'Kurz' was the name of one of the famous German climbers who perished on the North Wall of the Eiger in the 1930s."

Dr. Kurtz looked at me, waiting, without reply.

Me: "I am a mountain climber, you know. Long ago as a kid I read all the literature about the Eiger. 'Kurz' as I recall ended up hanging on a rope just short of reaching the rescue party."

Dr. Kurtz: "My family's name in Poland was Katz. My parents changed it to Kurtz."

Me: (After a slightly awkward pause.) "Well, I've just been wondering all these months since the stroke, and no one has been able to tell me, what is it that I can or cannot do now ...?"

Dr. Kurtz: "No one can tell you that, Karl. Every stroke is different."

Me: "For example, can I go climb a '14er'? No one says yes or no."

Dr. Kurtz: "We have our medical licenses to not lose, Karl. No one will tell you that you can go climb a 14er."

Dr. Kurtz and I smiled at each other. Five minutes into the 15 minute appointment it was pretty clear to me that the answers to my current dilemmas were not to be found in a doctor's office. Why hang around any longer?

I had already climbed all 54 of the 14ers in Colorado, some many times. Probably 130 peaks total. And in recent years I had found it sufficient just to get up into the high country for a nice hike to a lake or up to an above-timberline mountain ridge. To inhale deeply and luxuriously that pure air and to gaze at those wide high-altitude vistas. I knew well enough that I didn't need to climb any more 14ers.

It was really the loss of the professional part of my life that was nagging at me, not whether my mountaineering career was over. Before the stroke, I was still going strong. *"He is a math professor at the University of Colorado, and as per his chart, appears to be very high functioning at baseline despite his advanced age,"* the nurse had written flatteringly in my intake notes when I was admitted to the ER at Exempla Hospital. Now that part of my life was over. Completely over! The stroke had canceled everything professional.

Doctors tell us that most of our recovery from a traumatic brain injury, such as a stroke, will occur during the first year. In other words, my condition now is a fairly good measure of my future prospects. It's not that I'm not expected to make continued progress in the months and years ahead, for we know that the brain is quite "plastic". But we also know that the brain is not elastic and does not tend to bounce back quickly. Rather, the brain's process of making accommodations is slow and often subtle. Recovery is apt to last for the rest of my life.

I have made enormous strides in my recovery during the past year. My thinking is clearer, my synapses feel as though they're firing more quickly, my short-term memory has returned, and physically I am without any lasting impairment in motor functions or speech. These are all causes for celebration. It's easy to lose sight over time of the gains made when there are gaps that remain. And although I understand that I will continue to make further gains over time, I am aware that a complete recovery to my previous condition is not imminent.

The obvious conclusion to all these facts dawned on me slowly: It was time to retire from my position at the University. There was no further need to deny it. I calculated that my Sick Leave would run out in May, 2018. I would be 83 years old. This was an honorable exit age. So why not retire? That reasonable question begat another equally so: But what would I *do*? I had learned long ago that I like to have goals. And I like having achievements. What would they be? Staying alive was a new one. Second, write some books. Third, help my kids and my grandkids and my friends. There was plenty to do. I would be able to expend whatever energy I could summon up.

The poet Dylan Thomas famously wrote, "Do not go gentle into that good night. Rage, rage against the dying of the light."[1] But don't be a fool either. One definition of intelligence that I like is: the ability and willingness to recognize and accept new realities and successfully adapt to them. You could call this practical intelligence. I find it a lot more useful measure than something that can be determined on an Intelligence Quotient scale.

Life is given to us and death is unavoidable; but the in-betweens are really up for grabs, ever-changing along with our relationship to what each moment brings. Quite simply, the changed in-betweens in our lives, whether from a stroke, loss of a loved one or any other life challenge, are rich opportunities if we can learn to accept and grow from them. It isn't that I would have chosen to have a stroke. But that choice having been removed from my hands, the choice I do have, and now embrace, is where to go from here, one year post-stroke. And I chose to make the most of this life still before me, as it takes on a new shape.

---

[1]Dylan Thomas, "Do Not Go Gentle Into That Good Night," *The Poems of Dylan Thomas*, New Directions, 1952.

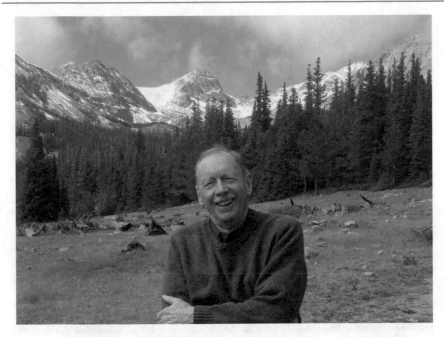

**Fig. 1** The author hiking in the mountains west of Ward, Colorado, near Brainard Lake, about 20 months after his stroke, 2017. Photo courtesy of Norm Nesbit

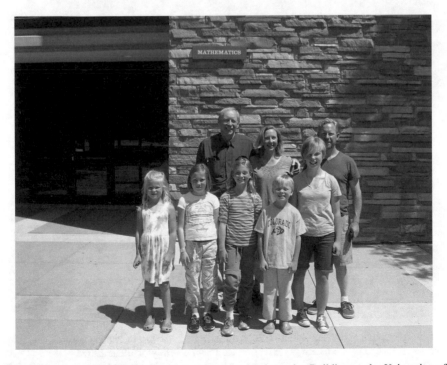

**Fig. 2** The author and his family on a visit to the Mathematics Building at the University of Colorado campus in Boulder, 2015. Photo courtesy of Cal Finch

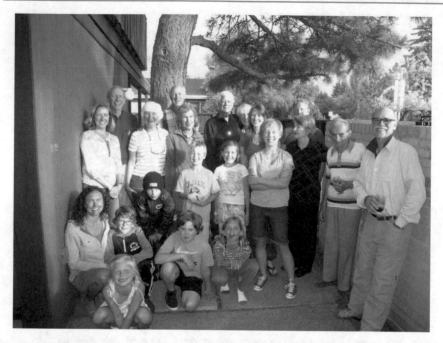

**Fig. 3** Family and friends gather with the author on the occasion of his 80th birthday celebration, 2015. Photo courtesy of Cal Finch

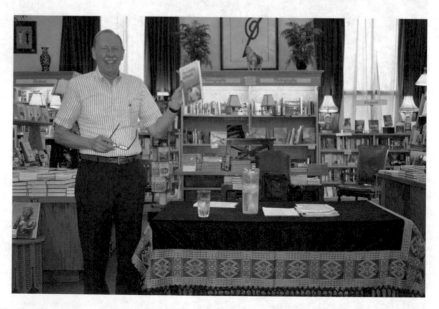

**Fig. 4** The author at the Boulder Book Store during a book-reading promoting his autobiography, *The Crossing of Heaven* (Springer, 2012), 2012. Photo courtesy of Jillian Lloyd

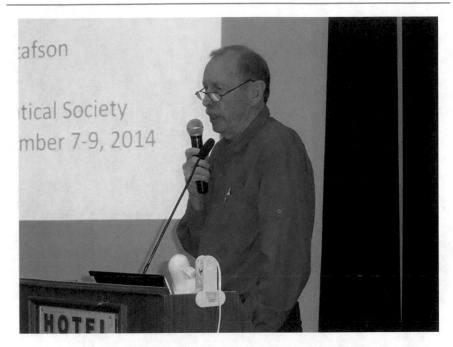

**Fig. 5** Author delivering the keynote lecture at the Hellenic Mathematical Society conference in Veroia, Greece, 2014. Photo courtesy of Ioannis Antoniou

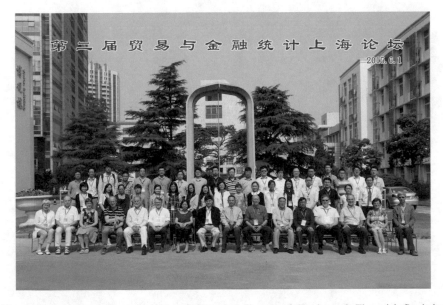

**Fig. 6** Group photo from the Second Shanghai Forum of Trade and Financial Statistics conference (SFTFS-2015), at which the author, front row center, was the keynote speaker. Also pictured is the author's friend Simo Puntanen, front row, 6th in from the left, 2015. Photo courtesy of Yonghui Liu

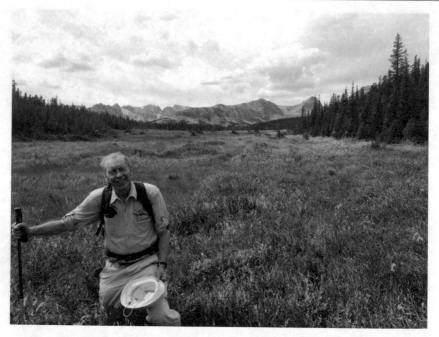

**Fig. 7** The author is pictured on a fall hike in the Indian Peaks Wilderness Area, near Ward, Colorado, 2015. Photo courtesy of Norm Nesbit

# New Reality

# 9

## …escaping limbo

The one-year anniversary of my stroke came and went, and as the weeks slid by, I became uneasy. What comes next? Although I had set some goals, still I was nagged by a feeling of listlessness. Was I fated to stay in this state of limbo, without a clear purpose, for the rest of my life? It was fine to declare to myself: "Accept your fate, Karl." But what did that really mean? What was to be my fate?

A life of sleeping, eating, taking walks, and waiting—for what I wasn't sure— seemed dull and flat to me. I am used to being productive! I need a purpose beyond that of mere survival. But one year post-stroke, with the attendant drama now behind me, I struggled to reclaim my life purpose.

One advantage was that I was in my home, and that required me to maintain it, as I have always done. A late spring storm brought several inches of new snow last night, which piled up in drifts, awaiting my snow shovel. Shoveling my own sidewalks has always been a great pleasure. It gets me outside and into the fresh air, and it gets my blood moving. It also appeals to my enthusiasm for daily goals. As soon as I finished my morning cup of Swedish coffee, on went my coat, hat and gloves, and I hurried outdoors to accomplish at least *something*. Clouds obscured the mountains to the west as I shoveled, but I took pleasure in knowing that they were there. The physical activity also cheered me. I mused, what if I had been paralyzed by the stroke? But how fortunate that I could still tackle a sidewalk full of snow on a frosty morning!

Getting in and amongst life in this purely physical and practical way this morning helped deliver me from my funk. As I continued to shovel, I gave myself a little pep talk: "Okay, Karl, you can consider some life goals, but they must be reasonable. The chief goal this second year is for you to learn to cope with your new reality."

After I returned inside, I warmed myself with a second cup of coffee and went upstairs to my office. For some reason, going upstairs in my house always lifts my spirits. The 600 sq ft upstairs is comprised of several rooms added to my house when my second wife and I combined families. Now the kids are all gone and the space has transfigured completely into one grand office. Sunlight streams in through windows on all sides.

© Springer Nature Switzerland AG 2019
K. Gustafson, *Reverberations of a Stroke*,
https://doi.org/10.1007/978-3-030-12862-3_9

On one desk next to my computer are some chapter drafts toward this book that I managed to write during the past year. I began this book as a therapy, trying to make sense of what happened to me during the stroke and in my recovery. The idea was to record events and impressions as they unfolded and were fresh, notwithstanding that my mind was not yet completely reliable. My editor Jillian had great patience and even greater tact in gently pointing out the various and occasionally very serious deficiencies in my efforts. At the same time, she encouraged me to keep writing, to write anything.

Now I wondered whether it was time to set some entirely new goals. Just jump in and start working toward them! Maybe I could climb Mt. Everest? Or go on a boat tour in Antarctica! Or do both. During the past year I have had the feeling that I must do something, anything, to counter the occasional bouts of depression that at times shroud my psyche. But I have also acknowledged that my physical energies are too low now to really jump into some such grandiose new adventure. The new reality is that I am alive, right now, still here. What a wonderful thing!

Today, rather than immediately sitting down and trying to write something, anything, or review a previous draft, I decided instead to just let my mind roam free, and allow it to guide and tune itself.

My thoughts went back to Tibet and to my wonderful trips to that high mountain kingdom. In 1994, in between my lectures in China, three of us drove in for seven days to Lhasa from the north. In 2001, I and another physicist and some Sherpas took nine students in from Nepal from the south and trekked for 10 days on the north slopes of Everest. How would I do now at an altitude of 18,000 ft? Ought I to try to seek out such strenuous high altitude again now? I think not.

My five trips to the Quantum Theory conferences in Sweden in the early 21st century then entered my mind. I had gone to the quaint and pleasant little village of Växjo in the southern Swedish highlands in 2002, 2007, 2008, 2009, and 2011. There I had greatly enjoyed discussions with the mostly European participants, many of whom I knew from the previous conferences. The dynamic Russian Andrei Khrennikov had built a world-class center for quantum mechanics conferences in Växjo, with a high tradition not unlike the famous Solvay Conferences in Brussels 100 years earlier. I was always welcomed as an Invited Speaker, with free choice of topic. In previous years, I had been able to present my thoughts and unique insights on Bell's Inequalities, The Born Rule, Elementary Particles, The Trigonometry of Entanglement, and Detailed Balance.

And it occurred to me that if I went again this year, I could present a summary of responses to my queries to top physicists over the last 20 years on how they think physically of "*fields*". Fields are a mathematical construct that can accomplish great things for you. And I definitely felt a physical field of an electrical nature when a lightning bolt knocked me unconscious in 1997 near a mountaintop in California. Presumably I was inundated with electrons. But I don't know what an electron actually is physically. And so far my queries indicate that no one really knows. A wonderful answer from one who had worked extensively and impressively both theoretically and experimentally was: "It's whatever I want it to be, a little ball, a wave, a cloud—it's whatever works for me".

But as I don't have a definitive answer either, how would such a lecture be received? From past experience, I would expect an appreciative few and many more who would gladly and fervently give me their answer, some with high emotion.

Then my thoughts went to Greece. I had lectured in Thessaloniki in 2011, 2012, and 2014. I could visit Ilias, my last Ph.D. student, who now works there in the business of remote surveillance and deep learning. I could chat about new encryption techniques with the brilliant young Fotios. I could enjoy visiting my wonderful colleague Ioannis and talk complexity theory with him and his students.

Maybe in another year, I concluded. My November 2014 Keynote lecture to the Greek Mathematical Society had been a high note. Let it stand. Besides, I have not traveled at all since the stroke and am not really sure if I can.

Think back, Karl, I remind myself: Your goal when you were younger was always to get back to Boulder, and to grow old in Boulder. And here you are! This is where you belong. It all worked out. Time to congratulate yourself!

\* \* \*

I have had no strong urges to go back to pure mathematics. I do have a favorite problem I think about occasionally, a very famous one, where I think I may have had an original insight. Once in a while I take out that folder. There is still a gap in what I know and what I need to know to go further. And right now, I don't feel like devoting my whole life's energies to pushing this endeavor to publication.

There are several other open mathematical problems that only I know and which I could easily share with new Ph.D. students. But taking on a new Ph.D. student is a multi-year commitment that I am in no physical or mental condition to make. Besides, I have already produced more Ph.D.s than anyone else in the University of Colorado Math Department. And I will no doubt be retiring soon.

I do like thinking physically about quantum physics, of which I have built up a lifetime's intuition. But I have no strong need to again jump into that highly competitive professional arena. Nor do I want to travel the world right now to defend anything I might publish.

In the last year I have been invited to many, many, international conferences, hundreds in fact. Some are bona fide, and some resulting from groups around the world trying to drum up business. I am quite content with my decision after the stroke to say no to all of them. I don't even go to Denver, 20 miles away, if I can avoid it.

I have consented, when begged by certain editors, to referee a few papers specifically related to my previous results and publications. I always inform the editors that, due to my stroke, I will not do any detailed left-brain analysis to check claimed results, and will rely instead only on my long experience with the issues.

My free musings bring me back to my conclusion that I may as well accept a coming retirement and try to write a book or two. The limbo I now feel myself trapped in at times, and which I view as so abhorrent, is the result of a physical change in the energies available to me. Fine! Let us get on with the new reality, rather than getting lost in the previous life.

\* \* \*

My inclination, throughout my life, has never been to dictate and pursue an outcome, like a super-salesman, but instead, to try to gauge the flow, and let it carry me. Although I have been willing to row upstream at times if the goal seems worth it, I prefer the poetry of, "*Row, row, row your boat, gently down the stream*". My boat hit a sharp rock in the form of the stroke, but it did not break apart, and I am still in it.

# An Early Rise

# 10

## ...to a different world

Summer came. As I was not teaching during the school year, its arrival was not noticeable to me. But summer came anyway. My daughter and her husband and three kids came to visit Grandpa Karl, as I am now known, for a week in June at my adequately large house. My son brought his two kids over. The five grandchildren were now 15, 13, 12, 10, 10, and I was struck with a realization that my role as the mysterious loved grandfather would not last forever. But this summer, fun and fellowship were had by the whole gang of us, in Boulder and in the nearby mountains. And then the rest of the gang departed and I was again alone in the house.

It is not unusual for me to awake at some early morning hour. Typically I get up, take a pee, and go back to bed. I have all my life greeted sleep easily, and since the stroke, even more easily. This morning felt different. We are having a cool and wet early August. There is still a lot of summer light. I considered, why not go out into the front yard? Maybe the morning newspaper is there? It was nearly 6:00 a.m.

I opened the front door and stepped out to a pristine morning. It was cool and the sidewalk damp under my bare feet. I have a five-foot high fence dividing my front yard into a small interior courtyard and a somewhat larger expanse of grass out to the street. I put my arms on the fence and gazed out at the world.

The four kinds of grass that continually fight each other for territory in that front expanse glistened heavily with dew. I preferred the native buffalo grass that had blown in of its own accord. It was thick and seemed to be slowly winning. It carried the most dew this morning. I also knew it to better survive the hot dry spells.

My gaze rose and detected a runner on the street beyond the large grassy schoolyard that provides my house with one of the best unobstructed mountain views in Boulder. Beyond the runner were the high and empty mountains of Boulder's unique and extensive wild parks system. The runner seemed to be in no hurry and was heading my way. I watched. He did not appear to notice me behind my fence and when he was not too far away, he abruptly reversed direction and headed into the distance again. It occurred to me that he could be my neighbor

© Springer Nature Switzerland AG 2019
K. Gustafson, *Reverberations of a Stroke*,
https://doi.org/10.1007/978-3-030-12862-3_10

Doug, who had run a four-minute mile when in college. I had observed over the years that my young, actually middle-aged, wonderful neighbors with their two boys tended to start their days early.

My eyes rose to the mountains beyond and detected a beginning alpine glow—or "alpenglow" as they say in Europe. In my youthful climbing days we would often see alpine glow when we were well into a climb above timberline on a peak in the high-country of Colorado. Today I was transfixed in my front yard, just watching the massive mountain cliffs slowly become a deeper and more beautiful pink.

Alpine glow signals the beginning of a good day. I felt good. Was this some kind of signal to me? Was I to enter a more energetic life after what had been a long eighteen months? A limbo that at times had led me to believe that it might continue forever?

I was a little surprised at myself, standing out there in my pajamas, and not feeling imprisoned within my usual post-stroke fatigue. What was going on? Why was I not frantically sliding back into the house and to bed? Would I crash later? I decided it did not matter.

Loud vehicle noises brought me out of my reverie. Voters had approved a large school-district bond issue. The school parking lot was being repaved. The school was also finally getting air-conditioning. No matter the national or international political moods, the American public liked to support their local schools. This great tradition remained intact.

A large piece of heavy equipment slowly backed off its long-bed transporting truck and entirely blocked the street. Six a.m. on a cool morning and workers and other equipment were arriving. I went out to the street and could see that there would be a big effort today on the main school parking lot. The smaller parking lot had already been paved.

My reverie was interrupted again by a movement to my left. I glanced that way and saw that it was my neighbor Anne. She had wandered out to check the extensive flowers in her well-cared-for front yard. Doug had told me that Anne loved her yard. I had noticed that Doug himself was not so often doing yard-work, but was often out with his boys on their bikes.

Such a nice, cool early morning. I drifted back toward my front fence. The sun was not quite up but we were bathed in the full light of dawn. I waved at Anne but she either didn't see me or pretended not to and slowly turned to head back into her house. Had she come out to check on me? One of her friends, a physician's assistant, had warned Anne after my stroke that I might not live much longer. And here I was, her 82 year-old neighbor, standing essentially motionless for 45 minutes on a cool wet morning outside his house, still in his pajamas and bare feet.

By now the sun had finally pulled itself up above the Eastern horizon as the Earth rotated, and the pink alpine glow was giving way to a bright morning illumination of the great mountain cliffs and the mountains themselves. Still more construction workers and equipment arrived. To be here at this hour, the workers who lived in towns miles away would need to rise at 5 a.m. or earlier. My own son did so every morning. Such was the real working world. Real America.

Still I stood there watching it all. The sun had fully hit the great rocks and mountains rising 3000 ft to my west. But where was my morning newspaper? I stepped out to the street again just as a small pickup truck rolled up with the driver's window open and I saw my newspaper deliveryman for the first time in my life. He had been extremely reliable for years, but we had not had occasion to meet. We smiled at each other as he tossed me the paper. He was not young.

Why was I not going back to bed? Why was I not dragging in total fatigue? Was it the cooler weather these past two weeks? Or was this the transition I had been hoping for, when my second life finally regained the energies of my first life?

I moved back behind the fence, grasping the newspaper in its protective plastic sack in my left hand. Despite the paralysis on my right side during the stroke, I was delighted during my recovery at how well my left side could do most things (even though I am right-handed). But after some weeks the right side began performing again and I now only remember the paralysis on those rare occasions when my right side seems to go slightly numb. Was it my willpower that had caused my paralysis to disappear? And if so, could my willpower also defeat my seemingly excessive need for sleep?

Finally I went inside and began writing this account. At 8 a.m. I prepared a light breakfast of buttered toast. Sitting at my breakfast table, I looked out and saw the sun's glow dimmed by large grey clouds, a high and dense mist that completely obscured all of the peaks to the west. There's a lot of moisture around this year, but the mists would burn off soon.

* * *

August 1 marked the passage of 18 months since my stroke. The neurologist had stressed the 18-month point as significant for gauging recovery following a stroke. I was sure it was a good average measure and that his intentions toward me had been genuine. But I was also sure that he knew as well as I did that I could continue to see improvements beyond that point. Each stroke is individual, as is each individual's recovery process. The neurologist's job is to treat the general, not the particular. I had not been satisfied with his somewhat impassive manner. Yet it had been useful to me. I was quite willing to take any useful advice and integrate it into my life. The advice was useful to me, but I also had decided to give myself another six months to assess my level of recovery. And now, 11 days later, I seemed to be experiencing some kind of wonderful transition point.

I decided to call my son Garth. I had not talked to him for at least a month. Not able to afford a house in Boulder, he lives in Erie, about 20 miles to the east. I had happily helped him buy a house there. He is a real working man in Real America. As manager of the parts department at a busy automobile repair shop in Boulder, he drives the 20 miles every morning to open his shop by 7:30 a.m., works till 5:30 p. m. and then commutes back home. One evening a week he goes to a local pool room after work, taking on all-comers. He plays to win and usually does.

"New Parts. This is Garth," my son announced into the phone.

"Hi, Garth. This is your dad. Everything is fine."

Silence. No immediate reply. So I continue: "I just called because I am up early this morning. And I feel good! This is the first morning since the stroke! The first time in eighteen months!"

"Well, that's good!" he replied. Garth is a man of few words.

"Anything new? When do the kids go back to school?"

"Well, next week we buy all the school supplies and then their schools start the week after."

"How about that roof repair?" I asked. His Homeowners' Association had been putting pressure on him to replace his roof.

"Well, I got some bids, including a good one, about $10,000. Farmers Insurance declined again to cover it. So I will change insurance companies."

"Sounds good." I replied, continuing. "As I told you, I will cover it. You know I think your house is a good investment."

"Well, its value keeps going up!"

I really like how he never asks for money, yet now accepts when I offer to provide financial help. I like to help. We understand each other. I am in the white-collar elite. He is a blue collar non-elite, in a capitalistic system which has evolved to favor inherited wealth and white-collar education, and which has almost completely deleveraged the real working population.

I looked at my kitchen clock: 9:00 a.m. For the last 18 months I have struggled to even get out of bed by then. Today I have already been up for several hours. I am writing away without exhaustion. Has the body changed its metabolism? Still in my pajamas, I am not bothered by the coolness of the morning. Why am I not collapsed on the sofa?

At 10:30 a.m. I feel small pangs of hunger. Why not shave, shower, get dressed, and head down to the shopping center for brunch? At this hour probably my favorite restaurant would be relatively empty. But when I get there at 11:00 a.m. it is jam-packed. Even the outside tables are all taken. So I wait for a table and am very hungry by the time I am seated. I order the special egg scramble, choosing the included sides of fruit cup and French toast. The meal goes down readily with two cups of coffee. Energized, I am soon bounding out the door for the five-minute walk back to my house to continue writing.

The day continues along like this. Occasionally I wander outside to survey the construction progress, then I write some more. The weather remains cool, which agrees with me. I notice little things, such as a very slight movement in the inner grass outside my window. I sit inside looking intently and then another blade of grass sheds a tiny drop of dew and raises itself slightly. This is new, to be so awake.

At 4:00 p.m. I decide to walk down to the shopping center again to another restaurant and grab a burger for an early dinner. On the walk back home, I see that all the construction workers and equipment are gone for the day.

Then it was time to convert all of my day's handwritten notes into an electronic form. I went upstairs to my computer and accomplished that by 10 p.m. It was time for bed, but what a great day it had been! Sixteen hours of steady energy and productivity: The first such day since the stroke. This gives me hope, and hope is so important.

# A Trip to the High Country

## ...lifting the spirit

I had not been up to hike in the Colorado high country since my stroke. As a lifelong mountaineer, my spirit is always lifted by heading up high and breaking through timberline into a wonderland of blue lakes, bordered by windswept ridges and soaring peaks. There is something about traversing wild mountain terrain that brings a religious feeling to me. I feel free, and closer to God. I have always taken to heart the inspirational words of John Muir: "Climb the mountains and get their good tidings".

In the year following the stroke, I felt the loss of this beloved pursuit keenly. But I had adopted a stoic and justifiable attitude of: "Be patient, Karl, you survived a massive stroke! Don't risk attempting any heavy hiking at high altitude."

Then 20 months after my stroke, my long-time mountaineering friend Norm called me with an invitation I could not resist. "It's late September, Karl," he said. "Let's go up to that place you call the 'the Crossing of Heaven' before the season's first big snow comes."

The Crossing of Heaven is the informal name that I gave to a particular passage high in the mountains when I was writing my autobiography [*The Crossing of Heaven: Memoirs of a Mathematician* (Springer 2012)].[1] One day near the end of that writing project, I snuck away for a day of cross-country skiing in one of my favorite high country places, where a remote traverse at timberline delivers one from high alpine woods to a lofty, open wind-scoured slope, framed by the dramatic high peaks of the Continental Divide. That day, skiing alone in that beautiful and magical setting, the name of my book seemed utterly appropriate for that place. And so it has stuck.

But I had only visited there in deep winter and on skis. Norm is 83 years old and no longer a skier, so a winter visit really wasn't an option. But he has been much intrigued by the idea of visiting the Crossing of Heaven he has often heard me

---

[1]My autobiography was primarily intended to record for history my writing the software for the world's first spy satellite in 1960. The title of the book, *The Crossing of Heaven*, was intended to connote how the Satellite Revolution had changed the world.

© Springer Nature Switzerland AG 2019
K. Gustafson, *Reverberations of a Stroke*,
https://doi.org/10.1007/978-3-030-12862-3_11

speak of. As I quickly reflected on the suggestion, I realized I had not been there myself for several years. And mountain snowstorms were predicted for later in the week.

"Let's go tomorrow," I agreed with enthusiasm.

The next day we drove west for about an hour from Boulder toward our destination. So far, there had been only a dusting of snow in the nearby high country. Most of the tourists to the National Forest had departed by now, but one road to a trailhead remained open, and we took a leisurely drive to a near-empty parking area at an altitude of almost 11,000 ft. From there, I estimated the distance to the Crossing of Heaven to be less than a mile. Arriving by this shortcut would not be quite as dramatic as skiing in for over three miles in deep snow, and thereby emerging into a high alpine winter wonderland. But Norm wanted to see the place now and so did I.

Donning our light daypacks, we set out on foot from the car for a few hundred yards and found the short trail leading to the Colorado Mountain Club ski cabin, which I knew to be about one half-mile from the Crossing of Heaven, albeit off-trail. But having only ventured there before in winter, I had no bearings of the place and immediately got us lost in the woods. As I sought to backtrack, underfoot were large boulders covered with a dusting of slippery snow and surrounded by dense underbrush. Norm hesitated. In recent years he has been having balance issues and, understandably, has become increasingly cautious about plunging into bushwhacking challenges. For my part, I noticed that my eyes were not focusing properly. Was it the altitude? The stroke? Perhaps dehydration? I drank some water and then spotted the ski trail a few yards to our right. From there it was easier going.

We hiked on in silence. As we drew nearer to our destination, we were surprised to find that the Forest Service had installed some impressive trail junction signs mounted about eight feet high. We saw a sign up ahead directing a left turn toward the old ski cabin. That trail would route skiers through timberline trees for about 50 yards, giving them protection from the sometimes hurricane-force winds. But as a result, they would miss the awe-inspiring views at the Crossing of Heaven.

We continued on, broke off trail for a bit—and then suddenly there we were, with the magical beauty all around us. Norm and I stood there solemnly, taking it all in. Two alpine valleys, one leading up to the dramatic cone-shaped Navajo Peak, the other to the sharp-pointed Mount Toll, appeared majestically before us. In our youth, Norm and I had each climbed those two high peaks. Almost 70 years ago now. We communed a little longer.

Norm then suggested we postpone lunch to hike another mile or so to try to locate the four little hidden lakes seldom visited by anyone. There is no trail to them. Several years ago we had unsuccessfully tried bushwhacking our way to them, but had encountered really difficult going. But we knew we had gotten very close to the largest of the lakes.

This time, as we moved down the trail, some grey clouds descended and enveloped us. A light rain was falling, but no snow yet. Soon we found our point of departure from our last visit and were both stunned at how impassible the bushwhacking looked now. With a sigh and a shrug, we reversed direction and headed back up the trail. Just as we entered the Crossing of Heaven, the clouds parted and the sun reappeared and we were treated to quite spectacular views. The mountain peaks and high valleys were now covered with a fresh coat of snow sparkling in the sunlight. We found a weathered old log to sit on for our late lunch in this high alpine spiritual place.

There was no wind. A Clark's Jay, a species of notorious high-altitude camp robber, fluttered into land at the end of the log to my right. I spoke to it in heavy terms, closing my pack and moving my food and belongings closer to me. Seeming unflustered, she politely hopped along the log toward me. As I munched my cashews, I finally relented and offered to share. One after another, she accepted the nuts from my hand. Rather than eat them immediately, she took each of her little food treasures and flew off to cache them somewhere in the bordering trees. The feast continued as Norm also fed her. Soon a larger Jay, probably her mate, came seeking his share. He was more aggressive and too late! But Norm and I fed him a few morsels before we closed our packs and prepared to leave. The female returned from the distant trees, fluttering a few inches in front of me, and hovering for several moments, as if to say "thank you". And then she flew away.

We took our time on the hike back down. There was no need to rush. I was aware that everything was just as it needed to be, just as it was meant to be. And then I understood that my journey through these past months has been much the same—leading me every moment to where I am right now. I felt at peace and completely happy.

# Time and Space

# 12

## ...choosing context

In the days and weeks following my stroke, my sense of time and space was jumbled and fantastical. It reflected a novel mix of actual events, imagined ones, and remnants from dreams, all within timeframes that were utterly malleable in my mind. For example, when my friend Jillian visited me soon after my arrival at the Boulder rehab, before they had even allowed me outside for a breath of air, I regaled her with an imaginative tale of my having just come back from a morning walk with my good friends Ioannis Antoniou and Ilya Prigogine. I claimed that they had surprised me with a visit and we had taken a nice stroll to the downtown Boulder post office, where I'd mailed some letters to friends. In reality, Ioannis was at home in Greece and not even aware of my stroke, and dear Ilya has been dead since 2003. However, they had both visited me in Boulder in years past and we had taken walks downtown, even if not to mail letters.

Perhaps I had dreamed or imagined the post-stroke visit from Ioannis and Ilya. And while I hadn't walked to the post office, the previous day I had in fact given my son Garth some items to mail for me. In those early post-stroke weeks, there was this peculiar blend of truth, fiction, and sliding time scales in my mind. My brain, it seems, had not figured out how to be fully present and clear in real time and space. And it would take some time for me to get there.

Our internal time clock is a kind of sixth sense, as I understand it. Our commonly referred to five senses of seeing, hearing, touching, tasting, smelling, are those of recording instruments. But an internal clock also is aware of the environments in which we find ourselves. The well-known example of jetlag stands out. Another is when we wake up moments before the time we've set our alarm clock for. How does the unconscious mind know exactly what time it is? It simply knows.

The 2017 Nobel Prize in the category Physiology or Medicine was given to the American scientists Jeffrey C. Hall, Michael Rosbash, and Michael W. Young for their discoveries of the molecular mechanisms controlling circadian rhythms. The three scientists used fruit flies to isolate a gene that controls the rhythm of an organism's daily life. This "biological clock" explains how plants, animals, and humans adapt their rhythms to be synchronized with the Earth, in order to successfully evolve.

© Springer Nature Switzerland AG 2019
K. Gustafson, *Reverberations of a Stroke*,
https://doi.org/10.1007/978-3-030-12862-3_12

Although the Nobel Laureates used fruit flies in their experiments, the results also explain how our human circadian rhythms regulate behavior, hormone levels, sleep cycles, metabolism. Our inner clock is set precisely to adapt our physiology to the different phases of the day. All organisms, including humans, operate on 24-hour rhythms that control sleep and wakefulness and physiology generally, including heart rate and blood pressure, body temperature, alertness, and reaction time. Our 24-hour day, of course, is just that of one Earth rotation. Our 365-day year is just that of one Earth revolution around our Sun. Our bodies have evolved in accordance with the specifics of our particular Solar System.

Animals seem to have a more acute sixth sense of time. They also seem to have a sixth sense of impending natural disasters such as earthquakes.

Billions of solar systems have planets and each has its own time system. Any life there will reflect those natural time systems. Beyond recording devices like eyes and ears, the survival of each species depends on an internal time sense.

\* \* \*

As a mathematician, I have watched, and at times been involved in, studies of what are called dynamical systems. Most of these are modeled as nonlinear differential equations that, for example, can produce chaos. Time is always viewed as a straight line. But I had long wished to emphasize that time itself can be an extremely complicated dynamical system. The opportunity came when I wrote (with co-author I. Antoniou) the paper *Financial Time Operator and the Complexity of Time* (Mind and Matter 11, 2013). I had been teaching a course on financial derivatives and was struck by how stock markets all over the world receive millions of buy and sell orders each second, each with essentially differing volume, and each based upon differing information sources. This is a good example of the inherent chaos and complexity of time.

\* \* \*

I have been fascinated as I rehabilitate from my stroke by the changes to my own time scales. They were all instantly scrambled by the stroke itself, which seemed to have an impact like an earthquake. And during the critical-care phase I did not have any time scales at all. During the rehab period, slowly I was retrained in time management: Here is your schedule for the day. It is your responsibility to get to your Speech, Physical, or Occupational Therapy sessions at their appointed times. I had to learn Earth time again to arrive at the dining room for my breakfast, lunch, and dinner. Gradually I became aware of the passing of time and then developed the strong urge to go home.

Now I am in the second year post-stroke. At this stage I find that my principal time scale for this, my second life, has settled on months rather than years. I am writing this in Month 21. The phases of day and night have less influence over me than in my old life. When I am tired during the full light of day, I sleep, and sunrise is certainly not my cue to rise in the morning. For an animal in the wild, such changes could be life-threatening. But in my case, the new time scales make it easier for me to adapt to the new realities of my second life. I take advantage of anything that helps me to cope. Species that do are the ones that survive. When I accepted that the old time scales were irrelevant in my new life, it was easier to digest the plain facts of my new identity. One crucial thing: I was lucky to have survived and entered a second life.

But how does one approach a new life, wherein the changes are so fundamental? From my studies of neural networks, I have come to appreciate the role of *context*, and I turned to that for understanding. More specifically, the role of setting (or even just imagining) a context, is incredibly helpful in mental processes. I wrote several papers with co-author Jakob Bernasconi where we showed how humans, by imagining a context, can reach conclusions that differ from those of machine algorithms. In my recent paper *The importance of Imagination (or lack thereof) in Artificial, Human, Quantum Cognition and Decision-Making* (Phil. Trans. Royal Soc. **A 374**, 2015), I point out the inherent weaknesses of computers in establishing context. They just grind away and try to win by brute force. Why should we humans give up our advantage? After all, we want human results, not machine results.

I urge you to think in terms of context as you proceed through your life on your own individual journey. Be sure to surmise in which context you find yourself at this moment: do you want to be there? If not, imagine a better context, and develop techniques to get there. For example, I have set some personal rules for a happy life and one of them is, "Go where you are wanted". Thinking of your life in terms of context will help you determine where you are wanted (and also where you are not wanted).

Now I find myself in this new context: Karl, you had a near-death stroke. You survived. Accept it. Live with it. My new space has a much lower energy, so I have adopted a policy of "do one thing a day". That is enough.

Context might also be geographic, a physical place. When a university in Switzerland wanted to hire me long ago, it was very attractive. Double my salary, half my teaching load, and Switzerland is not too bad a place to live and play. But my first wife vetoed the idea and she was right. I love Boulder and have always held fast to the high priority of remaining here. And as my life moved on, I realized that I did not want to spend my old age in a foreign country. I am American and I want to die in Boulder, in Colorado, with my ashes spread around the mountains here. I want the context of Boulder to be my final context.

I am so happy with my decision many years ago to keep my house, so that I would be comfortable here in my older age. Each afternoon, I slide onto the sofa in my family room with floor to ceiling windows and look out at Bear Mountain. I soon drift off to sleep, and an hour or so later I wake up, groggy but content in this new life context.

# Neanderthal Days

# 13

...intuition and reason

Here in post-stroke Month 22 I am dreaming and sleeping a lot and that always makes me wonder, am I getting better or worse? Also it's December, so the days are getting shorter now. With less sun I sometimes feel I must be like a Neanderthal—wanting to get up late and stay warm in my cave.

Long ago, when I was a boy, the official account of the Neanderthals was that they lost out to the Cro-Magnons (us). It wasn't spelled out exactly how they lost out. They were burly and tough but the implication was that they were not that smart, and after we arrived in Europe around 30,000 years ago, they quickly vanished. Reading between the lines, one could presume that the Neanderthals had been vanquished.

But even as a young boy, I was aware of the incompleteness of that account. How were they vanquished? Were they wiped out completely in battles, or did they simply retreat? And if so, to where? It just did not add up. But it seemed clear that the Neanderthal era, which had lasted hundreds of thousands of years, ended very quickly as the Cro-Magnons moved in with a superior culture.

Then evidence was discovered that in certain places, the Middle East for example, Neanderthal and Cro-Magnon tribes had lived side-by-side. Apparently, they coexisted peacefully enough. Immediately the answer to the puzzle was clear: They had interbred. Put another way, the Cro-Magnons had absorbed them. My close friends from long ago could attest that I would assert this interbreeding answer to the puzzle during my early years. That no one agreed with me, I still find astonishing. But my explanation did not fit with their image of what we humans are: We are not "cavemen". We are superior creatures. My assertion was met with politeness or scorn or tolerance, but nobody climbed on board with me.

Then DNA was discovered. Later scientists in Europe (Svante Paabo et al. 2008–2009) managed to extract enough Neanderthal DNA to show that those of European ancestry carry 1–2% DNA from Neanderthals. Sometimes even more. Apparently our immune system has benefitted from that DNA. No doubt there are other improvements.

My intuition had been right all along. The more attractive Neanderthal women undoubtedly were taken by Cro-Magnon men. The more attractive Neanderthal

© Springer Nature Switzerland AG 2019
K. Gustafson, *Reverberations of a Stroke*,
https://doi.org/10.1007/978-3-030-12862-3_13

men surely were seduced by Cro-Magnon women. I have been around, of course. Have those who could not see the merit of my intuition not also been around?

Aside from my having been right, I like this story because it illustrates the power of intuition over reason. Reason is based upon culturally accepted norms, call them axioms if you like, whereas intuition integrates across several reason-domains, with different axiom sets, and it also somehow better incorporates experience, even to the extent of tolerating contradictions.

As a young mathematician, I remember reading about the Intuitionists versus the Platonists. The Intuitionists would usually lose to the more easily digested arguments of the Platonists. At that time I too was caught up in the Axiomatic Method. Certainty and Absoluteness carry a lot of persuasive power.

## Logic and Reason

If you look carefully at mathematical logic, you will discover after several years of study, as I have, just how limited it is. The great virtue of mathematical logic is that it demands and provides consistency. But I have decided that consistency is not Reality. Very few real natural systems are consistent. And human nature is even less consistent. But everyone wants to believe in something. And because we want a clear formulation of that something, that becomes an axiomatic system.

One cannot prove axiomatically any of those choices we make in our canon laws. But our intuition can judge them and support them or not support them. In the end, even our axioms can depend on our intuitions.

## Experience and Intuition

I want to leave intuition undefined. Not only is it grander that way, but also I do not want to reduce it to a set of axioms.

I have angered some of my colleagues by arguing for intuition over reason, and experience over axiomatic proofs. If the attack on me becomes too pronounced, I tell them that they live in a black-and-white world, whereas I am living in a multicolored world. But I have become since my stroke more content with my differences from my colleagues. We have all had different life trajectories. Why should we be compelled to have the same beliefs?

## Imagination and Hibernation

Only in my old age have I come to see that I have a very active imagination. This has been a great advantage to me in creating new mathematics and new science. I want to leave imagination, like intuition, undefined. But I am sure every reader can imagine what he or she wants imagination to mean to him or to her. Or if some extraterrestrial creature is reading this, it can render its own interpretation.

I even wrote a paper on imagination.[1] A main point was that our imagination sets the agenda for the meaning in our lives. And a selling point was that computers and quantum systems have no imagination. (Hence, they always will be inferior.)

Now it is December, and I allow myself to sleep in every day. The idea is just to accept this 12-hour per night post-stroke sleep need and see what happens. The result is better morale. And the thought occurred to me: did Neanderthals hibernate? Is my changed mental state in any way a form of hibernation? The crowd may yell that of course Neanderthals did not hibernate. They were like humans, and we do not hibernate!

I don't know if Neanderthals actually hibernated, but they had to survive long glacial Ice Age winters. Surely they tried to conserve their energy and hunker down until warmer weather returned. In fact, it's nearly certain that our Paleolithic ancestors slept more when the days were shorter and colder—and that those genes may well be carried by us modern human *Homo sapiens*. Some researchers even suspect that it's encoded in our DNA to shift to a sort of "hibernation mode" as the days get shorter.[2] The idea is that less daylight causes an increased production of melatonin, which in turn produces an increased desire and need for sleep. Let me tell you, I seem to need more sleep as the days get shorter. Then as the days grow longer again, I seem to need less sleep. It feels good to think of this as a natural human condition.

## Sun and Soul

I have found that as one gets older and especially if you have survived a major stroke, you should go ahead and sleep as much as your body requests. You do not need to crimp on sleep as you were forced to do when raising your family or holding down a full-time job. You are lucky to be alive and your soul may want both sleep and sun.

As I started to become aware of my surroundings in the BCH Rehab hospital after the stroke, almost immediately I was asking my physical therapists, "Why can't we go outside for a walk?" It was late February and the sun was shining and my soul wanted the sun. Fortunately the therapists responded by taking me out on walks in the neighborhood, rather than keeping me room-bound on the hospital's fourth floor. I am convinced those walks did me enormous good. I don't recall any other patients in that fourteen-bed rehab unit going outside for walks. But I would have recommended it to them if they had asked.

---

[1]See *The Importance of Imagination (or Lack Thereof) in Artificial, Human, and Quantum Decision-Making,* Philos. Trans. Royal Society **A 374** (2015) 20150097.

[2]*See generally,* https://www.naturalnewsblogs.com/winter-hibernation-sad-may-normal-human-response/; http://www.dailymail.co.uk/health/article-94678/Tired-hungry-sad-Relax-youre-hibern ating.html.

My Paleolithic ancestors likewise would have enjoyed walking outside as the early spring days brought warmer temperatures and cheerful sunshine. Their souls would have been nourished as they strode out of their caves in rock or ice into the sun and they could look forward to the promise of living another year.

# Gratitude

# 14

## ...don't wait too long

To place Life within a context of *Gratitude* is a great secret that is best realized and conceived of by each of us in our own way. Like many survivors of harrowing near-death events, I too have come away with a deep feeling of gratitude following my stroke. But it is not just gratitude at having survived the stroke. It is more a deep feeling of contentment. I feel an overall sense of peace and now easily experience the joy of the simplest of things. I find myself grateful for many small events throughout the day. I love my life and the people in it. I wonder why others are not morle grateful for their daily lives.

## He Who Kept Writing Away

The concept of gratitude as an all-encompassing context from which to experience one's life first came to my attention in a one-page letter I received from my life-long friend and fellow mountaineer William Bueler. It was the fall of 2003 and Bill and I had been friends for 50 years. We first met when I was a freshman at the University of Colorado in 1953, and that Christmas break we had gone down to Mexico to climb the Mexican volcanoes Popocatepetl (17,400 ft) and Pico di Orizaba (18,700 ft). After graduation Bill disappeared into the Intelligence world, but later he reappeared in Colorado and we climbed many mountains together. In 1994 we rendezvoused in China where I was giving some lectures, and we found ourselves in Lhasa, Tibet, exactly five years to the day of the Tiananmen Square massacre in Beijing on June 4, 1989. On that five-year anniversary the Chinese government suddenly shut down Tibet and all routes in. We found ourselves stopped in Tuo-tuohe at 15,000 ft, on the Chinese-Tibet border, until we were finally cleared to depart. On the long road from China, we saw endless trucks filled with soldiers and no other traffic.

© Springer Nature Switzerland AG 2019
K. Gustafson, *Reverberations of a Stroke*,
https://doi.org/10.1007/978-3-030-12862-3_14

But such events were no deterrent to Bill, who was fluent in Mandarin and loved visiting China. One of his favorite places was Lijiang in the southern three river gorges province of Yunnan, and in the fall of 2003, he invited me to go there for a month with a small group. But I was busy teaching at the University then and had to decline.

Bill usually wrote detailed accounts of his travels and would send out copies to friends. But the letter that arrived following his return in late 2003 was nothing like his prior reports. It was a single sheet of paper, titled at the top: *Things I am grateful for.* The list began with his family, and continued with his world travels, and his many friends. He ended the note with a few lines declaring that he had been diagnosed with incurable brain cancer. I can still remember my shock. He died within months, in March of 2004.

A few weeks before Bill died, he sent me a copy of his latest and just-published book, *A Tibetan Solution.* On a sticky-note attached to the front cover was a handwritten note, in an obviously scraggly and labored effort:

*Karl*

*Despite the brain*

*tumor, I continue to*

*write away!*

*Bill*

Bill departed his life remaining productive in a way he enjoyed and in which he could still contribute. There was never any evidence of a trace of regret over his circumstances or fate. Instead, he approached it all with gratitude and good humor. At the time, I was struck by this and mused at the notion of approaching even the most challenging of fates with gratitude. This was something to ponder.

## She Who Cared About Many

At the other end of the spectrum in his life approach was my father. With four older sisters who doted on him throughout his youth, he emerged as a very self-centered individual. By the time I was born, he was a successful businessman who needed and loved a lot of attention. Then when I was fifteen, my parents divorced. My father remarried a woman named Helen, who was only seven years older than I. And although they liked each other, after a dozen years they too divorced. Next my father married a woman named Betty who had three daughters and had lived on the Olympic Peninsula of Washington; she could have been cast directly out of the movie *An Officer and a Gentleman,* which by the way was filmed there. With Betty providing four females to shower their attention on him, it was a good arrangement. But my dad had a drinking problem and they too divorced. However in his last year of life, they had remarried when she was taking care of his assisted living needs. Of course, she took virtually every penny of his estate.

When I went to Seattle for the funeral, afterwards Helen and her third husband invited me over to their house. It was a very welcome invitation and I greatly appreciated the good company before I was to fly home the next day. With my father's ego needs and heavy drinking, he must have been not easy to live with, but somehow he and Helen had remained friends after their divorce.

After Helen's third husband died she stayed in touch with me and would send me $50 on my birthdays with a cheerful note attached. Helen was just a nice person with no ulterior motives and she was the only person in my life to regularly send me money. I appreciated the thought and would keep her up-to-date on how things were going in my life. Despite her three marriages, Helen had no children of her own.

Then one summer day Helen and her very attractive niece who lived in Denver appeared at my door and invited me to spend the day showing them around Boulder. Her niece had just broken up with some Denver Bronco's football player (I don't follow professional sports) and it was clear that Helen was attempting to fix us up. We three had a great day in Boulder and I arranged a date down in Denver with the niece. The niece was extremely pretty and lived in a gated neighborhood and her home was full of dolls and stuffed animals. And she was probably still thinking romantically about her football player. After a very civilized evening I beat a retreat back to my rather pedestrian existence in Boulder.

Some years later I received a call from a lawyer in Seattle. Helen at age 84 had gone into the hospital for a rather routine checkup and had died. I was in her will. The lawyer went on to explain that Helen had left her home and her car to her male companion, but she had also made provisions for persons A, B, C, D, E, F, G, H, I, J, K, L, M, N, O, and P. "Karl, you are P," the lawyer announced. I laughed and thanked him for calling and said not to worry about it. He asked me if I had ever inherited anything and I said nothing from my parents, but my Aunt Leona had no kids of her own and had left me some money that I just passed on to my kids. The lawyer had known my dad and Helen a long time and continued, "Helen had some stocks and a coin collection so it will take a while, but you should be happy to write a receipt for the money when it comes. But you must promise me that you will spend it on yourself, Karl." We laughed and it did take a while, but I was surprised when I received a check for $18,000, and I did put it toward a new car.

I was grateful for Helen's beneficent thoughts toward me. It was not the money. I knew that she was just saying in her birthday cards, "Karl, I care about you." It was an act of gratitude. Since she had no children of her own, probably all those letters of the alphabet in her will were for nieces and nephews and stepchildren from her three marriages. She was just saying how much she appreciated all of us. My 3% was a statement of her gratitude.

Since Helen died, I always include $50 in the birthday cards to my kids and to all five of the grandkids. Just to let them know that I am grateful for their existence. One should not wait too long to understand the power of gratitude, not only toward others, but also toward oneself.

The natural question arises, why aren't we more grateful throughout our "first" lives? That is easy to answer: We are busy. We take so much for granted. We are only learning as we go along. We have family and professional duties that pre-occupy us daily. We don't want to just sit around being philosophers when real things need to be taken care of. The game must be played.

After a massive stroke or similar experience, especially if you are not young, the game no longer needs to be played, and in many respects, cannot be played. So we are benched, or maybe find ourselves in the audience. We are free to cheer on the others, and to marvel at the game itself. We are able to take the time to be incredibly grateful for the game, and to be grateful for having been in the game.

I have become very grateful for having been given the opportunity to participate in the game of human life on this planet. Moreover, after the stroke, I consciously feel the additional privilege of having been accorded this second life.

There are so many moments in which I feel deeply grateful that I cannot enu-merate them all. They include walking to the bus stop on a sunny or wintry day; seeing the aspens in their autumn yellow in the high country; slumbering on my sofa in my family room looking at the clouds gathering over Bear Peak; feeling the joy of learning in the eyes of a grandchild; walking in the same steps on campus now as I did 70 years ago from my parents' house in Boulder; going to my Class of 1953 Boulder High School reunion; getting an email from some mathematician or physicist in China or Europe or Africa asking me a question about one of my papers. How lucky I was to be asked to present four different Keynote addresses in Greece, Canada, and China in the 15 months immediately before being struck down by the stroke. How great it is to finally have a $70,000 new roof after having lived with leaks for 45 years, and how fortunate it was that the job was completed only in the month prior to my stroke. How my two kids Garth and Amy stepped up to the plate and handled my affairs when I was incapacitated for five weeks after the stroke. There is so much more, but I think you get the idea.

I saved Bill's sticky-note and his one page *grateful* letter. Like Bill, I have decided to continue to "write away." This book is an act of gratitude for my life.

## To Whom Do We Give Thanks?

More generally, a rather fundamental question has come up in my daily life. I keep finding myself silently saying, "Thank you". To whom am I speaking with this offer of gratitude? Is it the Great Spirit who receives my words? There is really no need to answer this fundamental question. The question belongs to the Cosmos.

# Two-Year Anniversary

# 15

…the big picture

My stroke at age 80 coalesced three critical life events: a life-threatening health crisis; involuntary retirement; and the onset of dreaded old-age infirmities. While each of these circumstances might be inevitable in the long run, they also each carry significant potential to produce a psychological crisis in anyone's life. In my case, addressing all three at once has been more than a little humbling and often overwhelming. As I reflect back over the two years since my stroke, I see that it has taken virtually all of my energy to navigate and cope with these simultaneous life challenges.

As I have found myself dwelling on these challenges, I also have remained aware of the importance of keeping them separate in my mind, even though they are intrinsically conjoined. In other words, the stroke and its aftermath was a total game-changer for me, beyond anything I'd ever encountered before in my long and fairly adventurous life. I had to grasp this fully in order to accept my new reality and eventually to go easier on myself and others. While the inevitable may have been forced on me, my acceptance of my new life and its limitations ultimately was voluntary. By choice, I softened. I have chosen to embrace the open future before me.

In the months preceding my stroke, I had given four invited conference keynote addresses. Professionally, things were going very well. I still enjoyed teaching my courses at the University. Physically, although I was aware of the gradual onset of old age, I was still doing yoga, hiking, biking, and climbing 14,000-ft peaks. I was sitting pretty and still sailing along.

And then very suddenly—as it often goes with these things—I found myself facing a drastically new set of conditions. So just like that, here it was, the greatest personal ordeal of my life.

I began writing this book to help myself understand and come to grips with the stroke and its after-effects. I started writing this chapter at the urging of my lovely editor who asked me to close with my personal insights about the challenges of these past two years. She knows full well that I am not an introspective soul and that this would not be easy for me. Nonetheless I persevered, and this evening a breakthrough insight came to me: Why should I not have a serious health crisis at

© Springer Nature Switzerland AG 2019
K. Gustafson, *Reverberations of a Stroke*,
https://doi.org/10.1007/978-3-030-12862-3_15

age 80? Why should I not retire in my 80s? Why should I not be growing old after 80 years? One of the chief challenges of my recovery, I would venture, has been in accepting the inevitable—not merely mortality, but change itself. That above all is what I have resisted, I suspect.

As with any personal trial, I have come to understand that a stroke should always be viewed within the wider context of one's life. You must not forget the Big Picture of who you are. Because the stroke, or any other personal or health challenge, is not *who you are*, and it is not and should not become your identity; it is simply an aspect of your life that must be dealt with. Events like a stroke, sudden retirement, and, yes, even old age, do not change the essentials of who you are.

Then there is my family to consider and my five grandchildren in particular. Ashley, my oldest grandchild, is turning sixteen and about to get her own car. My son works hard and steadily, but without much opportunity to increase his salary, so I pitch in for such items as appropriate. I also am very happy to contribute to the costs and benefits of university education for his daughters Ashley and Elizabeth when the time comes.

My daughter and her husband were college educated and single for many years, so they probably have accumulated more money than I have. But I have started equally funded college-savings accounts for her three children as well. I sometimes say a little prayer that Amy and her husband Cal can avoid incurring any debilitating illnesses and be able to finish the raising of their kids. If they could not, I would do my best to finish the job. This might seem ridiculous in view of my age, but we all should have good intentions, after all.

On the one hand, I never intended for this book to be a pep talk. But certainly I have discovered certain things that may be helpful to keep in mind if you are a stroke survivor (or, perhaps, anyone else). They are as follows: (1) Each evening, be sure to congratulate yourself for what you accomplished that day, even if it is just one thing. (2) Praise others in your life for what they do well, especially your family members and friends. (3) Thank everyone, the bus driver when you hop off, the pedestrian stranger who lets you pass on the sidewalk, and God or the Great Spirit whenever you feel moved to. Do this quietly, softly, but consistently. You may even thank yourself at times for doing the right thing. Let gratitude be your trusted guide through the challenges of each day. We generally have far more to be grateful for than we ever realize.

Today I am grateful for my survival and future ahead, and I am grateful for each of you, here reading this plainspoken story of my recovery.

# Year Three

**16**

## ...the future continues

It is now late February. I had intended to close this book with the preceding chapter, at the two-year anniversary of my stroke. Recently in considering this tale of my two-year journey, I had observed that Year One could be summarized as Survival, Year Two as Acceptance, and that Year Three is to represent my Evolution. Then it dawned on me that the future has arrived already, and it continues to unfurl itself before me. Year Three is here and now. I find myself counting my life again in years, rather than in months.

The reverberations that are my new life arrive like the waves on the shore of the lake in northern Minnesota where we would vacation in my long-distant youth: Not breaking like surf at the seashore, but rather, these strong freshwater waves are impelled by their own mass and insistence. And they are as inexorable as the sea.

A key question emerged as Year Three began: Would I ever return to the Mathematics Department? Although that question had often dominated my thoughts during the preceding two years, still I had never formulated any retirement plan. But two years of Sick Leave had weakened my resolve to return to the pressures of a full workload of research, publishing, teaching, and presenting international addresses, and I wondered if and how I could shoulder that load. For that matter, would the department even want me back? I feared that they would not. I feared that during my absence I had become obsolete.

The new chair of the Math Department is a friend of mine, and in years past in the evening he would sometimes knock on my door and invite me on long walks with him in the neighborhood where we both live. We spoke of mathematics and sometimes a little professional gossip, and it reminded me of my years in Europe where one often takes walks with colleagues. I had not seen much of Sasha since my stroke, but we had taken a few short walks. Then one recent night I was reading under a single lamp in my living room when I heard a knock at my front door. It was quite dark outside, but when I turned on an outside light, there was Sasha. I invited him in and we had a delightful conversation. I did not bring up the question of retirement and neither did he, but the feelings between us were as warm as ever.

© Springer Nature Switzerland AG 2019
K. Gustafson, *Reverberations of a Stroke*,
https://doi.org/10.1007/978-3-030-12862-3_16

A few days later I decided it was time for me to discuss my future with Sasha, so I called the department secretary and made an appointment. I opted to spend that whole day at the Math Department, intending to test out the waters. All the vibes were positive, somewhat to my surprise. Then in my meeting with Sasha, he encouraged me to return to teaching, at least for a year. A new hire had been teaching my favorite course, Partial Differential Equations, for three semesters straight now, and she could use a break, Sasha said. I had stopped by her office a few times in the two years post-stroke and I did so again, mentioning my possible return. She confirmed she would be delighted if I came back. All signs pointed toward my saying "yes" to this unexpected offer and open arm welcome.

Survival. Acceptance. Evolution. In Year One I had really wondered if I would keep on living for another year. In Year Two I had battled accepting my fate, resisted it, but had finally came to terms with what I could not change. Year Three, evolving into my future, had begun to seem more appealing to me, but I hadn't really known what that would look like. Certainly I had not guessed that it might involve a return to teaching in the Math Department! But neither had I ever ruled it out, and more and more, I had quietly been working on a few math problems on my own time. I had found that the interest and desire were still there, along with the returned ability.

Now, given the option to return to teaching, I found myself looking forward to it. And this was a revelation to me: I could still be of use to the department. It was okay that I did not have my previous energies, which had taken me all over the world for invited addresses, on top of my standard teaching duties. I already had given more of those addresses than anyone else in the department. I could now enjoy teaching without the additional load of all the preparation for those addresses, each of which essentially required my attaining new original research results too. So why not just be a normal person, I thought, with a normal work load?

In truth, I did not even hesitate to accept the Department's suggestion that I return to teaching. It simply felt right for Year Three of my continuing journey.

* * *

Beyond our own consciousness, there is the larger scheme of things. While it is essential that we carry ourselves through life with integrity, it is also helpful and even healthful to keep in mind a larger consciousness: The sweep of time and our place in it. If you are able to subvert your own ego, as for example you may accomplish in trained meditation, you might enter a state where you can comprehend a much more expansive picture.

The ancient Anasazi, for example, knew this. At their spiritual gathering place in Chaco Canyon in northwest New Mexico they designed an entire city based upon the solstices of our Solar System. Walls were laid out in perfect alignment with the points where the sun would rise and set on the shortest and longest days of the year. Other of their architecture took into account the maximal and minimal lunar cycles.

The Anasazi knew that they were part of the cycles of Time, beyond each individual's particular lifespan. And it is a nice thing, it seems to me, to see yourself as a part of the cycles of Time. We all live in reverberations of the Cosmos.

* * *

I have really enjoyed writing this book. I do hope it (or parts of it) will be useful or interesting to you. I leave you now to continue your life as I move ahead to continue mine. Let us keep going. And go easy, my friend.

Printed in the United States
By Bookmasters